This document is geared towards providing exact and reliable information with regard to the topic and issue covered. The publication is sold with the idea that the publisher is not required to render accounting, officially permitted, or otherwise, qualified services. If advice is necessary, legal or professional, a practiced individual in the profession should be addressed.

From a Declaration of Principles which was accepted and approved equally by a Committee of the American Bar Association and a Committee of Publishers and Associations.

The information herein is offered solely for informational purposes and is universal as so. The presentation of the information is without a contract or any type of guarantee assurance.

The trademarks that are used are without any consent, and the publication of the trademark is without permission or backing by the trademark owner. All trademarks and brands within this book are for clarifying purposes only and are owned by the owners themselves, not affiliated with this document.

Disclaimer

All erudition contained in this book is given for informational and educational purposes only. The author is not in any way accountable for any result or outcomes that emanate from using this material. Constructive attempts have been made to provide information that is both accurate and effective, but the author is not bound for the accuracy or use/misuse of this information.

Contents

INTRODUCTION 7

CHAPTER ONE..11

WHAT IS PREMATURE EJACULATION?........11

CHAPTER TWO 26

MYTHS ABOUT PREMATURE EJACULATION
AND ITS CAUSE 26

CHAPTER THREE 33

THE SEXUAL ENCOUNTER...............................33

CHAPTER FOUR..47

ORGASM AND THE DIFFERENT TYPE THERE
IS...47

CHAPTER FIVE..58

BODY SIGNALS FOR VOLUNTARY
EJACULATION..58

CHAPTER SIX..70

DIAGNOSIS AND MAJOR CAUSES OF
PREMATURE EJACULATION 70

CHAPTER SEVEN...86

DIAGNOSIS & TREATMENT METHODS.........86

CHAPTER EIGHT 119

HOW THE FEMALE BODY WORKS 119

CHAPTER NINE 137

FOOD & DIET FOR A HEALTHY SEX LIFE..137

CHAPTER TEN 158

ULTIMATE EJACULATION MASTERY 158

CHAPTER ELEVEN...175

FREQUENTLY ASKED QUESTIONS AND ANSWERS ON PREMATURE EJACULATION
....175

INTRODUCTION

Many men who have been faced with the problem of Premature Ejaculation (PE) in the past before the discovery of modern sex therapy and medicines have faced this problem without any hope of a cure in sight. Those were the terms then, and any man faced with such a problem stand no chance of finding a cure. Not because they had no money to get one, but because there was no cure or any form of remedy to this ego-shattering menace that they were facing. No one had the cure, and worse of all, no one understands how this sexual disorder came into being. Not until in recent times, all the doctors and therapists could do was to recommend certain ointments that do next to nothing and have psychoanalysis session with them that cost those men both time and money. It was both costly and ineffective.

However, it's not all gloom and doom for men who are faced with this disgraceful problem. Sexual medicine over the years has undergone tremendous improvement, as doctors and specialists now understand why this problem persists in men and why it does. New sex therapy methods are now able to cure over *90 percent of men* who climax too fast in the space an average of 14 weeks of treatment. It is now a different story when it comes to looking for a solution to any sexual complaint that a man or a couple could have. A sex therapist is now more confident as to what steps and medicine to take makes the man and his partner enjoy sexual life. Long gone was the time of uncertainties and haphazard treatment. Except for a few rarities, all it takes these days is a couple of weeks of specific treatment with the supervision of an expert.

After over a century of search by medical experts of the connection between psychology and premature ejaculation, I am of the opinion that it is now appropriate to refer to PE as symptoms of both organic and inorganic risk factors accumulated overtimes that's deserving of both medical treatment and more attention. From the medical space at large. Premature ejaculation is, in fact, a real medical need, a multidimensional disorder comprising of a dysfunction of the physical, sexual organ with psychosocial components. However, it's worth noting that its medicalization does not leave out the impact of psychological factors in its pathogenesis.

This book will be of great help to men having sexual problems of premature ejaculation, not only because it contains clearly outlined instruction that is easy to carry out, but it also comprises of years of practical experience in my several years of dealing with couples or single men. They can now reliably use the new techniques thoroughly discussed in this book to effectively get over this sexual problem and go on to enjoy their sexual life with their spouse.

A lot of scientific verdict points to the fact that, by carefully following the guidelines in this text, men who suffer from PE can get the treatment they have always been on the lookout for. However, there is a note of caution. There are certain rare cases, where after following the instructions to the letter, yet there is no significant improvement in your sexual stamina. Do not panic. No cause for alarm. The fact still remains that you are curable, and the next course of action might be to work closely with your therapist in order to make sure you are not making any profound mistake while following the guidelines. And in some cases, it might be a result of some deep emotional and psychological issues that are connected to your present state of mind that's preventing you from getting your healing. Those are all viable options, and they are preventable.

In order to get the nest out of this book, you have to come clean with yourself. Be of a clear mind and know that this is a perfectly normal situation, and with all the right decision, you will start enjoying your sexual life again in matters of weeks. Remember to help yourself, and be open-minded, by not giving up on yourself too soon. Put all hands on deck and work with professionals that will be of help to you; all you have to lose at the end of the day is your sexual problems. PE is treatable and you stand an even excellent chance working hand in hand with an expert to help you get through it. You've got this. Good luck.

CHAPTER ONE

WHAT IS PREMATURE EJACULATION?

At the moment, there is no uniformly acceptable definition for Premature Ejaculation, also known as Ejaculatio praecox (EP). Premature ejaculation refers to a quick and untimely expelling of semen, that makes sexual intercourse unsatisfactory for both partners. In most cases, ejaculation occurs before, during, or shortly after penetration (before or when entering the vagina of the partner) and during most of the sexual contact. The ejaculation occurs earlier than the man his partner wants, which means he experiences orgasm too early often with minimal penile stimulation.

Premature ejaculation often causes distress for couples. Many experts believe that premature ejaculation is almost always the result of anxiety or other psychological causes. Others think that the supersensitive skin of the penis may be the cause. Having sex less often than desired can make the problem worse, making man more sensitive. Premature ejaculation is rarely caused by a disease, although inflammation of the prostate gland, hyperactivity of the thyroid gland or a disorder of the nervous system can cause the disorder. This sexual dysfunction is common in adolescents, due to hormonal changes, which make them more excitable, but it can also appear in adults, in this case, it is mostly related to psychological factors, such as anxiety, fear or stress, for example.

Premature ejaculation is a term used to describe a sexual dysfunction in which the man gets the ejaculation very quickly without satisfying sexual intercourse for the couple. This often creates a burden on the partnership, which is often the trigger for consulting a urologist. Premature ejaculation indicates the loss of voluntary control of the ejaculatory reflex. Some scholars on this topic define it as the inability to satisfy the partner, in at least 50% of sexual relations, since ejaculation occurs before the full accomplishment of the partner, believing that she does not have any problem that prevents her from having orgasms. Premature ejaculation can also be defined as ejaculation that occurs less than 2 minutes after penetration or less than 10 impulses. Delayed ejaculation is another health problem and means a persistent failure of ejaculation, in the presence of a satisfactory erection, is the inhibition of the ejaculatory reflex.

By definition, premature ejaculation also means permanent or recurrent ejaculation with sexual stimulation before or within one minute after penetration into the vagina, the lack of possibility to delay ejaculation always or in most cases, and the resulting psychological stress, disappointment, and avoidance of sexual activity. Premature ejaculation is only considered a sexual disorder if the above criteria are met. The causes lie in a neurobiological phenomenon, which can lead to rapid ejaculation, and are not purely psychological problems.

The thing with premature ejaculation is that it is understood as an ejaculation that is perceived too quickly and happens against the will of the man. These men cannot control their ejaculation or cannot control it sufficiently. They feel that they cannot last long enough during sex because they climax too early.

FEATURES OF PREMATURE EJACULATION

There are various definitions of whether there is premature ejaculation or not. It, therefore, plays an important role in how the person concerned feels about the situation and what kind of suffering they are under. There is no clear limit and the sensation of the affected men or the partner "what is normal" varies is subjective.

In general, premature ejaculation is characterized by the following features:

- An ejaculation that always or almost always occurs less than three minutes after the limb is inserted into the vagina
- The feeling of the affected person that they cannot influence the timing of the ejaculation, or cannot influence it sufficiently
- Negative personal consequences, such as suffering, anger, frustration and / or the avoidance of sexual intimacy
- Inadequate control of ejaculation

15

- The pressure of suffering in one of the partners (regardless of whether heterosexual or homosexual)
- Reduced intravaginal latency (within one minute)

WHAT HAPPENS DURING PREMATURE EJACULATION?

The normal sexual response in men is a gradual process. It starts with sexual stimulation, penis swelling, and an erection. The phase in which this high arousal is maintained without ejaculation is called the plateau phase.

This is followed by ejaculation - usually in conjunction with an orgasm, followed by sagging of the penis. This can be graphically represented as a four-step cycle: arousal, plateau, orgasm (in connection with ejaculation), and regression.

In men with PE, the overall ejaculation process is shortened compared to the normal process. A strongly increasing excitement phase with a normal erection is followed by a shortened

16

plateau phase and rapid ejaculation in connection with an orgasm.

HOW MANY MEN ARE AFFECTED?

The most common sexual dysfunctions in men is Premature ejaculation. Studies have shown that about every one in three men is affected. The interesting thing is: only a few men have such a high level of suffering that they need therapy. We know from our own study collective that a maximum of 3 to 6 percent of the men affected want therapeutic measures to "come later."

Premature ejaculation is a health problem of multifactorial origin; that is, many things can be related to the presence of this alteration. The history of previous sexual intercourse, medication use, anxious behavior, and disorders such as depression may be related to premature ejaculation. However, psychological causes play a very important role and are closely related to the development of this disorder and should always be assessed and treated. Anxious men who present an episode of premature ejaculation will have a greater tendency to repeat this behavior because, with each sexual intercourse, they become more anxious and with greater psychological pressure to perform their role satisfactorily. Many evaluated cases of premature ejaculation show a great concern for men to provide sexual satisfaction until your partner's orgasm. This pressure will cause more problems. The diagnosis is clinical and depends on a careful survey of the patient's history. In most cases, the main complaint is the difficulty of satisfying the partner.

WHEN TO WORRY?

Time can mean absolutely everything in bed. If you're climaxing earlier than you and your partner would like, sex is probably not satisfying for either of you. Premature ejaculation can be frustrating, embarrassing, and cause discomfort in the relationship, often damaging the health of the relationship.

SEXUAL DYSFUNCTION

While it happens infrequently, it's not a cause for concern. However, ejaculation are often a dysfunction if you:

- Always or almost constantly ejaculates within a minute of penetration;
- unable to delay ejaculation during sexual intercourse for most of the time;
- You feel distressed and frustrated and tend to avoid sexual intimacy as a result.

HOW EARLY IS "TOO EARLY"?

Contrary to popular belief, the average man has an ejaculation after about five minutes of sexual intercourse. Naturally, however, individual differences can be disparagingly great. The symptoms of premature ejaculation are, therefore, rather a description of an ejaculation that is subjective to the attitude of the patient or his partner (she gets to determine how early is too early). In addition, patients report that they cannot adequately control the time of ejaculation. This is why it is important to develop the skill of maintaining control in order to last long enough to satisfy your sexual desire and that of your partner.

5, 10 OR 15 MINUTES?

There are various studies on how long the penis stays in the vagina before the man ejaculates. On average, however, men "come" after 3 to 8 minutes - depending on the country in which the scientists conducted their various studies. Many will now think: Our sex sessions last much longer! With this subjective assessment, many couples are completely wrong. This is shown, among other things, by a study of mine. We played a film for men and women showing a 5-minute sexual act. The astonishing result of the subsequent survey: the men estimated the length of the nude video to be 24 minutes on average, while their partners were just over 12 minutes in their assessment!

Premature ejaculation (PE) happens when a man regularly reaches an orgasm (or ejaculates) much sooner during sexual activity than what he or his partner would have desired. If this happens again or again, there is no reason to worry. But if this problem keeps recurring, it is important to see a doctor. According to the International Society for Sexual Medicine, premature ejaculation corresponds to ejaculation that always or nearly always occurs before 1 minute of vaginal penetration or that has had a significant and uncomfortable reduction in the time to ejaculate, often to about three minutes or less.

If so, don't worry: premature ejaculation is a relatively common problem. Estimates show that one in three men have this condition.

TYPES OF PE

The theme (like everyone that involves sexuality) is very broad, and therefore, there are different classifications for premature ejaculation.

There are 5 types of PE:

1. **Lifelong PE (primary)**, which existed when you first became sexually active that is from the beginning of sexual life. This kind of man lives with the total impossibility of prolonging intercourse whatsoever. The formal definition for lifelong PE is: "Ejaculation which always or nearly always occurs before or within about a minute of vaginal penetration, and therefore the inability to delay ejaculation on all or almost all vaginal penetrations, and negative personal consequences like distress, bother, frustration and/or the avoidance of sexual intimacy."

The lifetime is when the man faces the problem from its first sexual experience and is characterized by an ejaculation that occurs always or almost always before the sexual intercourse or within a minute after vaginal penetration . In addition, there is an inability to delay ejaculation in all or almost all vaginal penetrations, which can lead to negative personal consequences , such as anguish, discomfort, frustration, causing many men to avoid sexual intimacy.

2. **Acquired PE (secondary)**, which develops over time after you have had a normal sexual life, without ejaculation issues. This means it appears in the life of an individual who controlled well There is no fixed definition for acquired PE, but it is believed to share the same characteristics as lifelong PE except that it comes on later in life after a period of sexual normalcy.

Already acquired is characterized as man develops premature ejaculation after a period of normal sexual functioning , which is perceived one significant reduction in the time between penetration and ejaculation for about 3 minutes or less taking ac negative personal consequences such as anxiety, discomfort, frustration also causing many men to avoid sexual intimacy.

3. **Situational PE**: If it only occurs in a certain situation, for example, with a specific partner

4. **Variable PE**: occasionally experiences premature ejaculation. It's not a problem, but a variation in the man's ejaculation time

5. **Subjective premature ejaculation**: where there is a control time above the limit of two minutes, but the patient is very dissatisfied with the duration of intercourse.

The use of other techniques like perineal exercises always plays a complementary role in basic therapy and can be very useful in that it reinforces the individual's perception of the structures of this region

CHAPTER TWO

MYTHS ABOUT PREMATURE EJACULATION AND ITS CAUSE

Over the years around centuries ago, when the understanding of experts concerning the science of sexual conditions has not been fully developed, many myths about the issues that give to premature ejaculation and the circumstances surrounding it were passed around. Myths that were stated as a result of the belief of the time. So-called beliefs and opinions have formed the backbone of the perspective of people and experts alike toward the sexual condition. It is of absolute importance to debunk those rumors and separate the facts from the popular opinions that are devoid of a strong factual base.

POPULAR BELIEFS ON THE CONDITION

Contrary to previous popular belief, premature ejaculation is not a physical problem. Many are of the opinion that premature ejaculation is caused by inflammation or irritation of the prostate gland or the urethra; however, this has been debunked and it is now nothing but a mere fallacy that was passed around during the years when people have not fully understood the condition. And to make matters worse, there were awkward and uncomfortable treatment methods that involve injecting silver nitrate into the penile opening during those times. It is worthy of note that not any of the above mentioned physical conditions will ever be the cause of premature ejaculation.

One of the few exceptions to this is if the man is affected by a neurological condition known as multiple sclerosis. However, aside this very rare case, almost all case of premature ejaculation is a natural sexual condition, not one that is as a result of some physical condition the man is suffering from. Some are even of the opinion that premature ejaculation is related to hypersensitivity of the penis, not that this is totally refutable, but hitherto, there has been no single evidence to support this theory. To further reinforce this claim, a certain test carried out on men suffering from PE and those not suffering from the condition revealed that there is no difference in the outcome of the two sets of men. In this particular test, any correlation that circumcision might have on men as far PE is concerned is also disproved. The belief that getting a circumcision will make you take longer to come is baseless, and in no way will circumcision increase your time to ejaculation. Both circumcised and uncircumcised men experience premature ejaculation.

IS PREMATURE EJACULATION NORMAL?

It can be believed that PE only occurs in men who are sexually inexperienced because of the fact that their penis is still very sensitive. There can be nothing farther from the truth. While it cannot be uncommon for men who are just starting to be sexually active to ejaculate in a short time, this natural *early premature ejaculation* eventually fades away as those men continuously engage in sexual intercourse. To debunk this myth, both men who are actively engaging in sex on a regular basis and those who are just starting to have the experience can have this condition. Hence the above belief that only men who are sexually inexperienced have PE is not true at all.

PREMATURE EJACULATION IS ALL ABOUT THE TIME SPENT INSIDE HER VAGINA

During sexual intercourse, the most important thing is that both parties derive sexual satisfaction and pleasure. If, as a man during coitus, you are able to achieve penetration for eight minutes before orgasm, but your partners only need five minutes to reach climax, then you will be able to give your partner sexual satisfaction every time you have sex. In another scenario where a man can last ten minutes, but the lady needs at least fifteen minutes to orgasm, then, even though this particular man last longer than the first man, he is not able to give his partner the desired satisfaction, consequently resulting to sexual strife between partners. The time you spend during penetrative sexual activity before achieving satisfaction varies from one partner to another. A man might take longer to satisfy his partner while another might take little to make her climax. Other factors such as the mood of the lady, and how turned on she is contributing to the total amount of time you need to spend inside her before you can give here that multiple orgasms she has always been craving for.

PREMATURE EJACULATION AND YOUR GENERAL HEALTH

It is no news that premature ejaculation can cause relationship strain if your partner is not sexually satisfied, but in terms of your general health, PE poses no risk whatsoever and is not directly linked to any serious health conditions. The rare case might be if it is a result of biological or hereditary factors.

Premature ejaculation does not affect fertility if you are able to achieve both erection and penetration of the vagina. The semen will still be able to travel to the egg for fertilization so far you are able to penetrate your partner. However, if you reach climax before you get the chance to penetrate your partner, this might hinder your fertility, and you will need to seek the help of an expert to find a solution or compromise.

SOME MORE FACTS

Here I separate more facts from the fiction that's been circulating about this unpopular sexual condition. Separating fact from fiction:

- An estimate of 1 in 3 men suffer from premature ejaculation at a certain point in lives.
- Premature ejaculation is neither a sickness nor disease but a mere sexual disorder and notes that even the foremost sexually active of men can suffer from it.
- Premature ejaculation is a condition that's medically recognized by key health organizations such as the World Health Organization.

- Substances like wine, beer, and certain pills and medicines can lower inhibitions and heighten sexual pleasure – but abuse of them can cause male erectile dysfunction, the lack to orgasm, and early ejaculation.

- Lack of sleep could cause low serotonin levels within the brain, which triggers your body to ejaculate sooner.

- Masturbating before sex can increase the length of time it takes for a man to ejaculate.

CHAPTER THREE

THE SEXUAL ENCOUNTER

For individual men out there, the process of sexual encounters is quite different. Your erection is triggered by several factors working hand in hand to create a sensation in your body that enables the secretion of the right hormone to set the action into play. No wonder you get those embarrassing boners at the most awkward of the moment and have to take a breath for it to go down. It's perfectly normal. All these triggers by your Willy are aiming to get you a sustained erection that's needed if you wish to derive sexual satisfaction as well as satisfy your sexual partner.

The penis is not the main player here when it comes to sexual arousal and ejaculation. By having this crucial knowledge in your arsenal, you will be able to put to use the techniques that will be discussed in the latter part of this book to better control yourself and discover the sources that are feeding your excitement, hence your premature ejaculation. In individuals, the triggers responsible for PE are different due to the fact each person has a different past and experience. By recognizing your unique triggers, you will be able to identify the best treatment methods for you.

To further reinforce this fact, by carefully studying your triggers points, by the time you start to work with your therapist, all the methods and recommended treatments will make sense, and you will more relaxed knowing that you are the right pathway for recovery. The more sense they make, the more focused and determined you are to go the length and make things work to better serve your sexual life.

STAGES OF SEXUAL AROUSAL IN MEN

Sexual arousal in human beings is in phases. Women take longer periods to get *warmed up* than men, and this is nothing more than the fact that women are more emotionally drawn to their sexual partners while men, on the other hand, are more on the physical aspect of things. For the careful analysis of the various players involved in the arousal of the penis, we will look into the analysis carried out by William Masters and Virginia Johnson in the 1950s but has been developed over time. From the above analysis, it's clear that sexual arousal occurs in five different stages:

- The Situation
- The Turn-On
- The Cruising
- The Point of No Return
- The Climax / Orgasm

The perfect illustration to describe these stages before picking each one is that of an airplane on the runway trying to take off. While the plane (your Willy) is on the tarmac (The Situation) and trying to take-off (The Turn-On), the unique trigger points that are peculiar to each man comes into play to ensure a successful take-off. Once the plane is on air, the next stage is to maintain control and remain steady (The Cruising). At this point, it is important to let go of all hindrances or turn off and enjoy the ride as much as possible. After having to take the time to enjoy the ride for a moment, it is important to keep track of all key factors in order to be ready for safe landing (The point of no return) and land safely at your desired destination (The Climax). We will carefully dissect the intricate of the different stages:

THE SITUATION

The situation can be described as a variation of both time and place that presents itself the opportunity for you to have sexual intercourse, call it the mating opportunity. The situation is usually accompanied by the kind of trigger that you will normally find intriguing about the time of your place of sexual opportunity. This time or place of mating chance differ for individuals, it might be a planned date with your partner, or it can be a spontaneous event that leads to sex, probably with a total stranger or even with your partner when the idea of sex just presents itself to be a viable option. The fact that there are variations of this situation that can eventually lead to sex means there are a number of triggers that are associated with them. The earlier you are conscious of the situation the earlier you can easily pick out the triggers that can lead to premature ejaculation.

Some other common situational factors that can increase arousal are:

- The level of excitement your partner derives from the sexual encounter.
- The amount of time devoted to foreplay.
- The level of intimacy and attraction between partners
- The type of new sexual activity engaged.
- The type of sexual experience you have.
- The extent that the partner fulfills your sexual expectations.
- A new partner unleashes the beast in your Willy.

One thing that is usually important with all aspects of The Situation is that most of the triggers that will be responsible for PE in a particular situation, for example, *the kitchen quickie*, will be rather less potent in another situation such as planned sex in the bedroom. It is, therefore, pertinent for you to be in control and be always conscious of your erection and ejaculation; maybe you are in for a quickie or for a prolonged sex session. The PE situational triggers will always want to make you fall back into the trap of early climax, however as you will see in the following chapters by following the right approach, you will be able to control your penis and come when you actually want to do so.

To be able to master the technique for managing the situational triggers, you should take note of the following:

- Understand your state of mind
- Manage your level of excitement for each situation
- Know your body state and any hormonal imbalance
- Be conscious of your sexual prowess
- Apply the right therapy steps to get the best out of your Willy

THE TURN-ON

Both men and women get turned on in diverse manners. Men are more on the side of envisaging the physical attribute of a lady, and they can even get turned on by mere physical touch from their opposite side, while ladies need emotional intimacy and readiness of mind to get started. The attributes associated with turning guys on can be varied and peculiar to each man. For some men, it might involve heart pounding, heavy breathing, blood rushing, heat, an increase in muscle tension, and so on. Just as each individual differs, so does their response to sexual arousal differs. The main thing that is common here is the fact that they are responding to sexual stimuli from the signs they see on their partner.

Down there, Willy has got its own sign to show for sexual arousal as well. Signs such as swelling up of the testicles, tightened scrotum, slippery fluid lubricating the foreskin, and so on. This lubricating fluid is known as pre-cum and can be likened to the exciting fluid that secretes out o a lady when she is getting close to climax. As a guy, you should be able to differentiate the pre-cum and the actual cum, which signals the end of your sexual excitement. Pre-cum differs from actual come in that it is a lot less thick and is in the form of mucus that accompanies the sexual arousal stage and it actually reduces as you age. Only about 1/3 of men experience pre-cum as opposed to coming that every man experience to signal to climax. Pre-cum has nothing to do with PE, and you should be perfectly relaxed as it okay for it to occur in the arousal stage.

What Happen at the Penis Level?

Sexual arousal or turning on triggers the erection of the penis for more sensitivity, especially in the head and foreskin part. It helps to stimulate the other sexual sense organ to get ready for the next stage of action, which is *the cruising part.* However, to get every other part up to speed with the next course of action, which is sexual intercourse (penetration of the vagina), the erection of the Willy must maintain its erection and this can be a problem with men with weak erection or erectile dysfunction. The only way to get out of this hole and get in the groove for the next stage, the mind must be ready to let go of any psychological hurdle and embrace change. This condition is both psychological and physical, so in order to get rid of it, both the mind and the body must be in the game to catch any loophole and make the necessary change.

THE CRUISE

There is a period in between the point of penetration and the point of no return – the cruising period. The goal is to extend this period as long as possible for you to enjoy being inside of your partner. By extending this period, you are giving yourself the chance to reach the point where your lady can experience multiple orgasms. Ladies take time to get warmed up, and the longer you take to reach your climax and enjoy every inch of the penetration, the better your odds of getting her to climax. We've already talked about the perspective aspect of PE that involves getting your partner the required satisfaction. If both of you are able to derive sexual satisfaction in almost every session, then the issue of PE will not arise. PE steps majorly from the fact that the man comes before actually getting her lady to climax or as in some cases, the man comes even before penetration.

So a key technique that needs perfection is to get to enjoy the cruising moments and try to extend it for as long as possible. During the cruising period, your brain is releasing a lot of hormonal releases that motivate your sexual stimuli and creates an even greater sensation of sexual tension. As you cruise along, you are riding on the wave of your rising sexual arousal, however, to make this last long in order to result in orgasm, you need to get rid of any form of mental blockage that might stand in the way of your sexual satisfaction.

As the tension builds up, you are in for a flight or fight mode, where you either take charge of proceeding while enjoying the ride or you succumb to your overexcitement and let it ruin your ride, ultimately leading to premature ejaculation. The standout contributors to this scenario are anxiety and stress. If any of these creeps into your sexual life, you are in for a struggle in your relationship. You have to let go of any form of mental tension that will cripple your sex life.

The opposite of stress and anxiety are passion and excitement, and you must ensure to have them be the mainstay of your cruising stage. Passion and excitement build up sexual tension in a good way that leads to great sex. What you should look out for and try to avoid is overexcitement, as this seeks to put you out of control, and when you are not in control, Premature Ejaculation is bound to happen. Not taking charge, makes the brain to bombard you with hormones that creates electrochemical reactions that move you from the cruising stage to the point of no return in no time at all, and ultimately PE.

We need to talk about the issue of youthful exuberance that robs young people of the ability to be mindful of their excitement level when in the cruising period. It is a known fact that about

30% of men develop a degree of control at some point in their sex life and don't have to worry about this issue any longer. However, they themselves are not aware that they are exerting this sort of control. What they did know is that at some point, they no longer have to worry about their youthful exuberance. Those who are not able to let go of their youthful exuberance on their own accord need to be guided by professionals to achieve control and have a quality sex life.

THE POINT OF NO RETURN

The point of no return, as the name implies, is that stage when you are totally in descent mode and ready to crash. Most of your reflex action in this period is majorly focused on getting that gush of semen out of your penis into your partner's vagina far in as possible. You might find yourself gripping her tightly to ensure she gets the whole deal of secretion coming out of you, or as in some case, you experience an even greater contraction to push the semen out with so much force as to go a long reach inside of her vagina.

This stage is where all the process responsible for emission takes place. The semen travels a great deal from the testes by a continuous wave of muscle contraction where they are transported from the epididymis to the prostate. The muscle contraction is to give the semen enough push / force for its transport inside the tubular organs.

THE CLIMAX

The climax is the expulsion phase and is basically about advancing the semen through the urethra and out of the glans for a push out. The pelvic floor and the bulbospongiosus muscle does a lot of background work in this phase. Accompanied by the gushing power of the tubular muscles, the pelvic floor and the bulbospongiosus are responsible for the shooting-like manner (or dribble-like manner) with which the semen passes out the penis glans opening.

You wouldn't take notice, but an average orgasm involves 10 to 15 contractions. The semen, however, gushes out at the second contraction, and subsides afterward, followed by a feeling of pleasure and relaxation. Your blood pressure goes up; your heart rate rises; your breathing becomes deeper and heavier.

THE SEXUAL ENCOUNTER AND PE

Not only is premature ejaculation robbing your partner of maximum sexual satisfaction, but it also reduces the amount of pleasure that you derive after you come. The longer you stay in the cruising mode, taking control of your excitement level, the higher the level of pleasure you derive from orgasm, since you are able to accumulate a high level of fluid before the climax. Premature ejaculation is robbing you of such a level of pleasure.

CHAPTER FOUR

ORGASM AND THE DIFFERENT TYPE THERE IS

You only know what an orgasm is after you've had one!" The experience of orgasm can vary from 'a sneeze from below' to an ecstatic peak. How do you experience an orgasm, and does it always feel the same?

WHAT IS AN ORGASM?

Earlier, we talked about the stages of sexual arousal, what to do about the 'orgasm gap' (with heterosexual sex men almost always come, and women who to a lesser degree squirt). But what is an orgasm? An orgasm is described as a peak experience of intense excitement and pleasure, accompanied by a changed state of consciousness, involuntary movement of the pelvic floor and sexual organs, and an intense feeling of satisfaction and bliss as a result. Have you ever experienced this? An orgasm is often experienced as ecstatic when there is both strong sexual arousal and many physical symptoms.

No genitals, muscle contractions, or specific sexual behavior are mentioned in the definition of orgasm. Why? Because orgasms always vary. Every person experiences it differently, and each time it can feel different for the same person. That is because the context is always different.

We know that orgasms can arise through stimulation of genitals but also through stimulation of the anus, thighs, breasts, or earlobes. They also occur without physical stimulation: in your sleep, while you are training, when you are fantasizing or just like that. Every orgasm can feel different: fine, ecstatic, spiritual, irritating, like a sneeze, deep or superficial, short or long-lasting. A specific context can lead to clitoral, vaginal, g-spot, or anal orgasms.

DIFFERENT PHASES

Men often describe an orgasm more based on physical sensations and women more based on the feeling that they get. This is because the feeling in women is less concentrated on one physical sensation than in men. Nevertheless, orgasms are not very different in men and women. You are in the first phase of cumming when you have the feeling that ejaculation (or ejaculation) or orgasm can no longer be stopped (point of no return). Then you come to the second phase where the feeling of cumming is determined by muscle contractions of the pelvic floor. In the male, contractions of muscles in the semiconductors, seminal vesicles, and prostate provide a 'pumping' sensation. In the woman, all muscles in the area of the vagina, urethra and anus contract, as well as the uterus itself.

My Little One

Popular websites and TV shows talk about the amount and types of orgasms you can experience. Is it one, or are there perhaps 15 types of orgasms? Because all structures are so interconnected within the pelvic floor and sexual organs, it is impossible to distinguish between different types of orgasms. Regardless of how and where the exciting stimulation takes place, an orgasm always results in the same physical reaction. For example, it is wrong that women still often make a distinction between clitoral and vaginal orgasm (Masters & Johnson, 1966)! The clitoris is so large that it can be stimulated from many sides, including vaginally. So what they call a 'vaginal cumshot' in the media is basically just a clitoral cumshot. Moreover, do not worry: for three-quarters of women, penetration sex is not enough to get rid of it. Matter of the right stimulation through masturbation, fingering, and / or oral sex!

FACTS ABOUT MEN'S ORGASM

It starts as a small stimulus, builds up - sometimes slowly, then again very quickly - and ends in a wave of pleasure that engulfs you. Yes, the pleasure of an orgasm is great. But because we - of course – already know what it feels like as a man, I would still like to remind you of some facts about male orgasm.

1. His G-spot

Do you not know where hubby is most sensitive to his penis? We tell you his most irritable places down under. The frenulum, which lies just below the 'mushroom-shaped' end (its glans), is a small, thin tendon that connects the glans with the foreskin. The perineum, the soft spot between his balls and his anus. His prostate, which can stimulate you manually. How do you do that? By massaging the perineum or (for the daring among us) by going into the anus with a finger and stimulating his prostate. It sits at about 5 centimeters and is a gland the size of a walnut.

2. Short and powerful

A 10-minute orgasm? This won't happen to a man. Men's orgasm takes only about 5 to 22 seconds at most. A short but powerful burst of emotions filled with an intense height of pleasure.

3. Fake it til you make it

Yes, men also fake orgasms. An estimated 30 percent of men have already pretended. The reason why those men faked their orgasm varies from individual. But it still remains the fact that men fake orgasm, the same as with women.

4. Little delay

Anyone who thought that men would always release their 'crap' when they cum is wrong. Sometimes, men do not ejaculate at all, or that only happens a few seconds after their orgasm. This is always possible before they reach the point of no return, after which there is no turning back.

5. Do-it-yourselfer

Two minutes or less. That is the time when 75 percent of men cum when they masturbate. Sex researchers Masters and Johnson concluded this. Moreover, they discovered that it is almost impossible for men not to get ready when they are stimulated.

SEXUAL ORGASM

An impending orgasm in the man leads to the swelling of the testes, and the acceleration through the cremaster musculus to high in the scrotum. The orgasm is caused by irritation of nerve endings in the penis, especially in the area from the frenulum to the scrotum, and to a lesser extent also at the edge of the glans (penis opening).

Orgasm in a man is usually accompanied by ejaculation. Physiologically, this consists of rapid rhythmic contractions of the prostate and muscles at the base of the penis, whereby the sperm stored in the balls are pushed out via the urethra. The duration and intensity of the foreplay can influence the orgasmic sensation. It is also possible to have a dry orgasm without ejaculation. This often occurs in children in puberty who do not yet produce sperm but are already masturbating.

The orgasm normally lasts between 3 and 10 seconds. It is usually, but not always, a very great pleasure. After an orgasm, a man usually needs a rest period before he can be brought to a new high again. Depending on the person and his age, this rest period can vary from one minute to more than half an hour. Stimulation of the penis during the rest period can be very unpleasant or even painful.

INVOLUNTARY ORGASM

Orgasms do not always take place voluntarily. Sometimes they occur with minimal unintended stimulation, or spontaneously. The best-known example is the wet dream, in which a person gets an orgasm during his / her sleep during a mostly sexually tinted dream. Certain activities can also trigger an orgasm without the person having intended it. Examples are horse riding or cycling with constant pressure on the genitals and certain gymnastics exercises. Certain medicines can also have spontaneous orgasms as a side effect. Sometimes this can lead to shame or an aversion to the activity that led to orgasm. Someone who is involuntarily sexually stimulated can get an unwanted orgasm.

FAKE ORGASM

Boys and young men often indicate that they have more than 1 orgasm per day, through masturbation or achieved by a partner. This decreases with age, though. For women, the number of orgasms seems to be less of an autonomous need: it is more determined by the presence and quality of the relationship with a partner. The inability of women and men to get an orgasm is called anorgasmia. If an orgasm is feigned to the partner, a fake gas is called. Both men and women sometimes use this to increase the pleasure of the other or to complete the sex session.

With coitus, 30% of the women get to climax regularly, while 90% of the men get an orgasm. This will be the by sexologists' orgasm gap or orgasm gap mentioned, a variant of the gender gap. Broadening sexual acts can bridge this gap

WET DREAM

A wet dream is the spontaneous ejaculation of a man during sleep, sometimes accompanied by a sexually tinted dream. It is a variant of an involuntary orgasm. The wet dream can occur at irregular times, usually during REM sleep. Wet dreams are most common during puberty or early adulthood, but can also occur later in life. Men can wake up during a wet dream or simply sleep through it. Wet dreams may be more common in boys who do not regularly masturbate or have sex.

The first ejaculation takes place in about 13 percent of the boys in a wet dream. Boys who have their first ejaculation during a wet dream are usually older than boys who have the first ejaculation through masturbation.

DRY ORGASM

A dry orgasm is an orgasm of the man without an accompanying ejaculation. A dry orgasm can occur if one is just on the edge of an orgasm and can be repeated so that the man - just like the woman - is capable of multiple orgasms at that moment. In dry orgasm, the man has yet to get to the point of no return. Hence he is able to prevent himself from climaxing. But when he does reach orgasm, he experiences a greater level of pleasure and more volume of semen gushing out of the penile opening. Sometimes there is an ejaculation, but one cannot see this. This is the case if the sperm goes through the bladder in the wrong direction, retrospermia. Another cause is nerve damage from diabetes mellitus.

CHAPTER FIVE

BODY SIGNALS FOR
VOLUNTARY EJACULATION

FOUR PHASES OF ERECTION

"I wonder why men can get serious. They have a long, delicate thing going up and down on their own. If I were a man, I'd always laugh at myself."

There are four levels of erection. For you and your partner, these are probably the easiest identifiable signs and the easiest to use to always be aware of your level of sexual arousal.

The first phase erection (stretching and padding) looks like a normal soft penis. There is no externally recognizable evidence of arousal or sexual arousal, but we call this a first phase erection because you are well aware of the sensation in your genitals. They start thinking about or fantasizing about sex. You want to touch yourself or your loved one or be touched. Sexual intercourse is not possible in the first phase, but you will probably think and visualize it.

The second phase erection (swelling) is a partial erection. A second phase erection begins to rise, but it is not a direct greeting. You can have sexual intercourse with an erection in the second phase, but this requires a "smooth entry." If the input is smooth, you or your partner manually insert the lingam (tantra for the penis) into the yoni (tantra for the vagina). Lubricate Lingam and Yoni with saliva, vaginal fluid, or a suitable lubricant (preferably a water or silicone-based lubricant). Stimulate a soft penis until the second phase erection by rubbing the penis with your hand on the vagina or with fellatio and then inserting the penis manually with your hand. A second phase erection is sufficient for sexual intercourse, but it is unlikely that your partner will be completely satisfied.

Phase three (full erection) is upright and saluting. Some men will ejaculate in the third phase, but ejaculations are much more common in the fourth phase. A third phase erection is completely sufficient to offer your partner a fully satisfying sexual relationship, but your partner's enthusiasm for climbing a fourth phase erection wildly is undeniable. The main advantage of an erection in the third phase is that a man can fully engage in active sexual intercourse without having to worry about the overwhelming urge to ejaculate. Most men can learn to maintain an erection in the third phase while successfully postponing ejaculation for longer periods of time, like for hours, not minutes.

Level four (rigid erection) is very proud and an unforgettable sight. Often referred to as "stiff," seeing some women can lead to climax. As Mark Twain said, "The penis is more powerful than the sword." Since the lingam is full of blood, an erection in the fourth stage is hard, notably more difficult than an erection in the third stage. It is also very hot and can make the color lighter or darker. The danger is that, for most men, an erection in the fourth stage means that ejaculation is unpredictable, perhaps imminent. Sexual control requires you to change or stop what you do and your erection to decrease. This is necessary if you want to prolong sex for a period of hours.

ERECTIONS COME AND GO

Normal sex is like a firework rocket. The climb is fast, followed by a violent explosion and a waterfall back to earth. A man can go through all four stages of erection in five or ten minutes (sometimes less!), Culminating in the ejaculation of sperm, which is ejaculation and abruptly ends intercourse. This is really shit, without sex, but based on that kind of initial experience (which is enhanced in Hollywood movies, where an entire love scene can be shot in less than 60 seconds). Men and their partners begin to believe that a man receives and maintains a single erection during every love session. Obviously, if all intercourse takes less than 30 minutes from start to finish, it is possible to obtain and maintain a single erection, and there is no reason to doubt it. On the other hand, a sex master usually prolongs sex for a period of hours - four or more. It is not uncommon for Tantric and Taoist masters to sleep twelve hours or more together. It should also be clear that no one could or would not want to get an erection for hours. With male sexual control, there are periods of sexual intercourse that begin and end during the period of sexual intercourse. does not exist hours of sexual intercourse with hours of the active collision. This is one of the foremost common misunderstandings about advanced free party practices. This misunderstanding is based on the false assumption that sex is a sexual relationship and does not take into account the countless other ways in which lovers come together in an ecstatic sensual / sexual / spiritual union. An erection is a cardiovascular event, which means that the lingam hardens when blood is collected and lasts only as long as that blood remains. Blood is the carrier of oxygen and hormones in the tissues of the penis. Oxygen is consumed during active sex and, while hormones are chemically converted, waste material accumulates in the penis and in the surrounding tissue. If the old blood is not removed, the man is sexually exhausted and is at risk of premature ejaculation due to this tiredness.

In the male sexual domain, men have their erections reduced every thirty to forty-five minutes. As the erection wears off, the used blood comes out of the lingam and takes all the waste with it. With the resumption of active sex after a period of rest, the man regains his erection when new blood penetrates the penis and provides a vital supply of oxygen and hormones. He is fresh, strong, and masculine again and can endure long enough to keep up with his partner in sexual stamina without having to exert himself superhumanly. Once you understand that maintaining a single erection for hours is neither desirable nor possible, you are psychologically prepared to allow and let go of the erection to actually promote it. You wouldn't fall into the trap of worrying about why a man goes limp during intercourse. On the contrary, it is an important skill in male sexual control - that is, the sexual master skillfully masters his erection, knows when to soften his penis, and when to stimulate another erection. This knowledge is an important key to preventing the common problem of fear of failure that affects so many male lovers. While men sometimes mistakenly treat women as sexual objects, they treat men as successful objects just as often, with the direct result that they also treat men as sexual performance machines.

OTHER WARNING SIGNS OF EJACULATION

When you approach the point on your sexual arousal scale where ejaculation begins if it becomes unpredictable, your body may warn you with one or more of the following situations to draw:

- Your breathing can become fast, irregular, irregular, or irregular.

- You can make sounds, including groans from animals, moans, and screams. Unless they are intentionally quiet. The natural tendency is to be noisy.

- Muscle tension, contraction and tension are a clear sign of unpredictability Ejaculation. The tension is visible in all or part of your body. You can pinch your fists together, pinch your lover too hard, and bend your stomach muscle and put on your buttocks.

- Due to increased blood flow in the chest, neck, face, ears, and nose, washing can take place in the upper body.

- Your testicles come closer to your body, and your eyes are glassy just before ejaculation.

PRE-CUM

Pre-cum is nature's lubricant excreted by the lingam to lubricate the yoni during sexual intercourse. A man can continuously secrete pre-sperm for a period of hours from the end of his penis, as long as he remains excited to a phase three or phase four erection.

The popular silicone-based lubricants are copies of the feeling before the hose very smooth. Urine has a clear odor, while pre-sperm is odorless. The sperm is always cloudy, while the sperm is completely clear. If there is something turbidity with this separation, you know that you are almost approaching a full one ejaculation.

ALARM SIGNALS FOR INTERNAL EJACULATION

The internal signals from the body are the most subtle indicators, but also the most reliable when it comes to how close you are to ejaculation. When you're very good at noticing it, you'll notice you always have the option to continue using it to release or delay ejaculation and transition to higher energy levels. In other words, at this point, ejaculation will be almost entirely voluntary.

Achieving this level of awareness requires that you go through your sexual arousal process many repetitions. Fortunately, this is an extremely enjoyable task!

The prostate is found under the bladder and surrounds the urethra leave the bladder. The urethra is the tube through which urine and sperm flow from the body. The prostate exhales a thin, milky fluid that lubricates the skin urethra and prevents infections. The most important function of the prostate is the production of most liquids in semen, including those that feed and transport the sperm.

When sexual arousal reaches a certain threshold of intensity, yours becomes the sympathetic nervous system that sends the reflex centers of the spinal cord to start the ejaculation reaction. Usually, however, this whole process is involuntary, but you can voluntarily carry it out with the type of training described in this guide.

Internally in your genital area, you have smooth muscle tissue. Another name for smooth muscles is involuntary muscles. What will you do with the exercises that we suggest in this manual, to take on a voluntary character and be able to control your involuntary smooth muscles? Once the ejaculation reaction has started, it cannot be stopped. Smooth muscles at the base of the penis contract every 0.8 seconds gushing out about 5 ml of sperm with 300 million sperm from the tip of your lingam in no less than five powerful thrusts.

During sexual intercourse, the hot sexual energy accumulates at a high intensity in the genital area with special concentration in and around the prostate. The ejaculation reaction involves violent contractions of the vas deferens (i.e.the tube for transporting sperm from the testes to the prostate) and contractions of the testicles prostate that adds prostate fluid to the sperm and completes the mix you produce known as sperm. The urethra filling activates the internal muscle tissue that causes it.

Rhythmic contractions in the surrounding organs, including the erectile tissue of the penis. At the same time, most men (who haven't learned to relax), let the pelvic and abdominal muscles with powerful pressure movements. The result is an enormous increase in internal pressure, which greatly produces sperm.

When the hot sexual energy builds up with excitement, you get to the point where it feels like the orgasm is just starting. This feeling is undeniable - it looks exactly like the start of ejaculation. When you have slowed down and are. If you are very careful, you will surely feel it. That feeling gives you enough notes to be able to change what you do and allow the energy to reduce to a more manageable level. You can get on with sex and rebuild yourself to another peak of energy.

CHAPTER SIX

DIAGNOSIS AND MAJOR CAUSES OF PREMATURE EJACULATION

HOW IS PREMATURE EJACULATION DIAGNOSED?

Numerous medical societies have defined premature ejaculation (ejaculatio praecox, in short: EP) differently. A distinction needs to be made between lifelong (or primary) and acquired (or secondary) premature ejaculation. A conversation with the doctor is enough for him to make the diagnosis, along with a thorough physical examination and a little more in-depth conversation about the health history of the affected personnel.

If the patient experiences premature ejaculation and, at the same time, problems with maintaining an erection, the doctor might order some blood tests in order to check the testosterone levels in the bloodstream.

In the first case, the problem has existed since sexual activity began. In the second case, there was a period in which the time to ejaculation was experienced by the man as sufficient and satisfactory. The diagnosis for Premature Ejaculation PE or "Ejaculatio praecox" is based primarily on the information provided by the people affected. During the conversation, the doctor should, therefore, ask the patient in detail about their sex life. The open question about sexuality and satisfaction with sex life makes it possible to get important information as part of the anamnesis.

In heterosexual men, the time between inserting the penis into the vagina and ejaculating should be addressed. If the said time is regularly less than a minute, one speaks by definition in connection with the psychological stress of early ejaculation.

A distinction should be made to be sure if it is a primary ejaculatio praecox, i.e., it has always been this way or a secondary form, i.e., it only started occurring in recent years. The distinction is important because the therapy options can change accordingly. Other diagnostic procedures, such as laboratory tests of blood or urine, are used primarily to rule out underlying diseases (e.g., prostatitis , etc.) that can cause ejaculatio praecox.

For an examination, you can contact a urological or family doctor's office. The doctor then asks about the average time to ejaculation and how often it occurs too early, how stressful the problem is and whether the ejaculation can be delayed. Further examinations are only useful if there is suspicion of a medical problem.

The diagnosis is made if

- there is almost always an unwanted ejaculation within a minute of inserting the penis;
- premature ejaculation has occurred for more than six months;
- heavily burden the premature ejaculations and

- no other diseases are responsible.

Medically speaking, it is not premature ejaculations, though if;

- they occur only occasionally.
- you have been sexually abstinent for a long time. Then it is normal to be aroused faster at the beginning and to climax earlier.
- the time until ejaculation is in the normal range, but is felt to be too short.

The examination also examines other options that could affect the time to ejaculation. Inflammation of the prostate is considered a possible risk factor. If the prostate is inflamed , the inflammation should be treated first. Signs may include frequent urination and painful urination.

Premature ejaculations can sometimes be the result of erectile dysfunction - for example, when a man hurries because he is afraid that he can no longer maintain the erection. Then the main problem is erectile dysfunction, not premature ejaculation.

Addressing premature ejaculation is an essential step, which often involves a lot of effort. To diagnose EP, the doctor conducts a detailed anamnesis interview, which should include not only the physical condition but also the honest response to social and sexual life. Possible medication intakes (e.g. psychotropic drugs) are also essential . Furthermore, the doctor clarifies whether it is a primary or secondary (acquired) EP. Possible underlying diseases are included in the diagnosis (e.g., Inflammation of the urethra). It is also crucial whether the man concerned actually has an EP or whether he only suspects that he is "sick" due to incorrect assumptions regarding the "right" time of the ejaculation.

The affected man should have the following examinations performed for complete diagnosis and therapy:

- Biothesiometry (for measuring nerves)
- EMG (to measure the pelvic floor muscles)
- Doppler duplex sonography (for measuring the four vessels of the penis)

- Examination to determine the composition of the erectile tissue
- Blood sampling (examination of various hormonal parameters)

PREMATURE EJACULATION AND ITS SYMPTOMS

The first symptom of early ejaculation is when ejaculation happens before expected. However, this problem can happen in all sexual situation, including masturbation. The main symptom is the inability to delay ejaculation for quite a moment after penetration.

However, this problem occurs in all sexual situations, even during masturbation. A lot of men feel that they have symptoms of premature ejaculation, but the symptoms don't meet the diagnostic criteria for this sexual dysfunction. Instead, these men may experience natural variable premature ejaculation, which includes periods of rapid ejaculation as well as periods of normal ejaculation.

Doctors usually classify PE into two categories, mainly primary and secondary.

Primary premature ejaculation is categorized by problems identified throughout the patient's life. Look:

- Difficulty holding an erection with less than a minute of penetration
- Inability to delay erection during sex
- Frustration, Stress, and the act of avoiding sexual intimacy with the partner.

In secondary premature ejaculation, on the other hand, the man manifests exactly the same symptoms as the primary ejaculation, with the difference that the symptoms were not always part of his sex life. Men who experience this type of premature ejaculation have had satisfactory sexual relations in the past and manifested the problem for some reason.

Psychological and biological factors can also play a role in premature ejaculation. Although many men are embarrassed to talk about it, premature ejaculation is a common and treatable condition. Medications, psychotherapy, and sexual techniques that delay ejaculation - or a combination of them - can always help improve sex for you and your partner.

CAUSES OF PREMATURE EJACULATION

Do you hear that term, and are you all bothered? Well, it is to be expected; after all, premature ejaculation is nothing more than the inability to control ejaculation during sexual intercourse. Because it is considered taboo by most men, many guys take too long to seek medical help - and that only makes it worse.

Research has yet to establish the exact causes of premature ejaculation, but it has already been linked to health conditions such as prostatitis (inflammation of the prostate), anxiety, and other psychological issues. Some experts say that there is a genetic relationship to PE, while others believe in a chemical imbalance or changes in the sensitivity of the receptor in the brain of some men. Many men with premature ejaculation feel ashamed, anxious, depressed, and concerned about pleasing their partner. Single men sometimes avoid new relationships because of the stress generated by the condition. In young people, the cause is usually related to anxiety and inexperience of the sexual act. Treatment is basically performed through sexual psychotherapy (which may be behavioral) and pharmacotherapy.

All men, especially young people concerned about premature ejaculation, should be encouraged to see a urologist. There are several treatment strategies available that can help men delay ejaculation time. The exact cause of early ejaculation is not known. Although it was once considered exclusively psychological, doctors now know that premature ejaculation involves a complex interplay of psychological and biological factors.

It is noted that one in four men suffer from this disorder at least once in their lives. However, what turns the event into a "problem" is the frequency with which it happens. If the dysfunction becomes routine, you need to seek medical help and know that, in most cases, premature ejaculation is caused by psychological issues. Want to find out the main causes? We separate a list:

PSYCHOLOGICAL FACTORS

Some psychological factors that seem to cause premature ejaculation are:

- Anxiety
- Depression
- Sexual abuse
- Erectile Dysfunction
- Relationship problems

- Early sexual experiences
- Unsuccessful love relationships
- Distorted body image or shyness
- Preoccupation with premature ejaculation
- Professional problems that may cause excessive concern
- Fear of getting the partner pregnant or not fully satisfying her
- The use of some medications, such as psychotropic drugs, can cause premature ejaculation.

BIOLOGICAL FACTORS

Some biological factors that can be related to the problem are:

- Genetic factors
- Thyroid disorders
- Abnormal hormonal levels
- Hormone levels above normal
- Abnormal ejaculatory system activity
- Neurotransmitter levels above normal
- Genetics and hereditary conditions

- Infection in the prostate and urethra
- Abnormal levels of brain chemicals called neurotransmitters
- Damage to the nervous system caused by traumatic experiences or surgery.
- Diabetes (patients with diabetes may have problems with their sexual potency)

RELATIONSHIP PROBLEMS FACTOR

If you've had satisfactory sex with other partners where early ejaculation has occurred infrequently or not, it is very possible that interpersonal issues between you and your current partner are contributing to the problem.

SOCIAL PRESSURE

The man is constantly asked to be the perfect lover, the stallion, the good in bed, and the catcher. Men spend a lot of time under pressure, which can trigger dysfunctions such as premature ejaculation.

RISK FACTORS

Some factors can facilitate the occurrence of premature ejaculation, which are explained briefly below:

- **Erectile dysfunction**: This is the problem of having or maintaining an erection. You may be at increased risk of PE if you infrequently or consistently have difficulty getting or maintaining an erection. The fear of losing your erection can make you rush consciously or unconsciously into sexual encounters. An isolated episode of sexual impotence can affect you psychologically and take over your subconscious, and this will affect later relationships. If erectile dysfunction is recurrent, premature ejaculation may become even more acute.

- **Stress and Anxiety**: emotional or mental instability limits the ability to concentrate and relax, which can lead to the occurrence of this problem. Health issues, such as heart disease, can increase anxiety during intercourse and cause premature ejaculation. It is difficult to escape these two points that affect health in several aspects of the society in which we live. Sex logically is a mirror of your emotions, and if you are under great stress or experiencing an anxiety attack, it is very likely that you will have frustrated sexual intercourse and premature ejaculation. So, see a doctor to combat these symptoms.

DESPERATION FOR PENETRATION

Sometimes men forget that penetration is only part of sexual intercourse, and the act of having sex involves several other senses, touches, gestures, smells, and tastes. By keeping the focus only on penetration, the pressure on it can increase and, consequently, anxiety as well. So try to focus on other points in the relationship and forget about penetration a little, you'll see that everything will flow more naturally when you worry about the moment as a whole.

COMPLICATIONS OR CONSEQUENCE OF PE

Premature ejaculation can put considerable stress on the man, the partner, and thus the respective relationship. Reduced self-esteem, avoidance behavior, as well as stress and tension, can intensify the symptoms and cause other problems, such as erectile dysfunction. From physical point of view, there are no negative effects to fear. What does premature ejaculation do?

Premature ejaculation can put a significant strain on the relationship between a man and a woman. The man often has the feeling that he is experiencing little satisfaction or that he does not feel the ejaculation. Sometimes it becomes difficult to maintain an erection or a loss of sexual arousal. This is often due to an excessive effort to delay ejaculation. The man is so busy thinking about "technology" or avoiding movement that the fun of the sexual encounter is completely lost. Often, therefore, the "foreplay" is extremely shortened by the man, so as not to become too excited himself - this often results in a lack of excitement in the woman. This can result in a painful, unsatisfactory sexual contact for the woman result - without orgasm. In many cases, this results in a significantly reduced number of sexual contacts - up to the complete abandonment.

CHAPTER SEVEN

DIAGNOSIS & TREATMENT METHODS

TREATMENT OF PREMATURE EJACULATION

This problem, Premature ejaculation is a common sexual problem for men, occurring in 30 to 40% of adult men. It can reach men in all age groups, in a certain period of life. It is important in these situations that the community health agent builds a good relationship with the user so that he can have "openness" and confidence to talk about his problems. These cases should also be referred to as the health team doctor to continue the investigation and treatment.

There are various ways to prevent premature ejaculation. Which of these is the most suitable depends on the underlying causes of the condition. In addition, it should be clarified whether the development of the pelvic floor muscles is possibly too low and whether the nerves on the penis are too sensitive. This can be measured with a so-called biothesiometry. In addition to oral medications that change the composition receptors in the brain responsible for ejaculation, there are various options that are individually tailored to men to delay premature ejaculation. A distinction is made between non-drug therapy and drug therapy.

Also, the involvement of the partner is often the focus of non-drug treatment. Simply approaching the problem together leads to success in some cases and supports all further measures positively. This can also minimize the pressure to succeed (e.g. first step: sex without sexual intercourse). The drug approach primarily (only) treats the symptom as such. Surgical treatments cannot currently be recommended. It is, however, important to explore the causes of sexual disorder before undergoing therapy since premature ejaculation can have various causes, both organically and psychologically. The psychological component plays a central role, even in the case of underlying organic disorders. Which treatment option works best for affected men depends on the underlying cause. Therefore, you should definitely let yourself be examined by a specialist.

In principle, sex therapy is particularly useful when dealing with the problem of ejaculation praecox; experience has shown that many affected people seek a quick solution, which is why it is often offered alongside the medication. Other drugs, such as the use of PDE-5 inhibitors, local anesthetic ointments, opiates, etc., are possible, but the best results have been described with the SSRIs. At the same time, with the latter therapy options, you have to point out to the man that these drugs are off-label applications and that the preparations are generally not approved for them.

Whether and how to treat premature ejaculations is a very personal question. There are various options for treatment. Certain techniques are designed to help control ejaculation better by deliberately delaying it. One possibility, for example, is to repeatedly stimulate the penis until shortly before the climax and then to stop. There are also medications can extend the time to ejaculation somewhat. There are oral agents and anesthetic agents for application to the tip of the penis (glans) . Both can have side effects.

HOW CAN PREMATURE EJACULATION BE TREATED?

After differentiating into primary or secondary ejaculation praecox, the therapy options should be discussed after intensive consultation with the person concerned. The only approved drug for treating PE to date is dapoxetine, a serotonin reuptake inhibitor (SSRI), which has shown a significant extension of IELT in many studies. This medication must be taken one to three hours before sexual activity.

Sex therapy is also a powerful treatment that aims to give men or couples more self-confidence and to ease the fear of sexual "inadequacy." Another goal is to concentrate less on ejaculation and to live sexuality more diversely. Relationship problems can also be addressed if they play a role.

WHEN DOES PREMATURE EJACULATION NEED TREATMENT?

An affected man's first step should be an open conversation with a partner. The (suspected) problem should be discussed openly in order to clarify whether it represents a problem for the couple with regard to the experience of shared sexuality. If both partners experience sexual intercourse as fulfilling despite a rapidly occurring ejaculation, there is no need for action. However, if it is confirmed that premature ejaculation is a burden on the common sexuality, an introduction to the urologist may be useful.

Premature ejaculation can be treated depending on the cause. Therapy can be medicinal, mechanical, and psychotherapeutic - but can also consist of a combination of several therapy options if a possible underlying disease is included.

WHOM CAN I ASK?

Ongoing problems with premature ejaculation should be discussed with a urologist. The general practitioner can also be contacted and can make an appropriate assignment. Doctors from various disciplines and psychotherapists can be involved in the diagnosis and therapy process.

Sexual problems - like premature ejaculation - are still a taboo subject. They can be associated with a high level of suffering. It is believed that not all affected men seek medical help. Having identified any of the symptoms or causes listed above, it is important to seek the advice of a psychologist or psychiatrist . They can help you deal with problems like anxiety, stress, or depression that can contribute to low performance during sexual intercourse.

If your relationship is affected, the first step is talking about the problem. A good psychologist or sex therapist may be able to help. Schedule your appointment today and lead a happy and healthy sex life. After all, sex is life!

NON-DRUG MECHANICAL THERAPY (BEHAVIORAL MEASURES)

There are several methods that helps to delay ejaculation that does not include popping pills but mainly specially designed techniques to achieve results. Non-drug techniques such as the start-stop technique and the squeeze technique attempt to delay ejaculation and these behavioral measures are most effective when used in addition to other medical treatments. However, different methods work best for different individuals.

With the start-stop technique, the penis is stimulated, and the stimulation is interrupted just before the ejaculation (or just before the feeling that the ejaculation is inevitable). After the excitement has subsided, it starts again. With the squeeze technique, the sexual act is also interrupted shortly before the climax and pressure are applied with the thumb on the glans base of the penis (area of the glans, foreskin ligament) to reduce the blood volume in the corpus cavernosum (penile swelling body) and to delay ejaculation.

Targeted pelvic floor training/potency muscle training

The ejaculation reflex is triggered not only by the ischiocavernosus and bulbospongiosus musculature but also by the corresponding nerves. If these structures are very well trained, the man can prolong the sexual act through special training. You can find training plans here

Stop-start technology from Semans

With this technique, the penis is stimulated until shortly before the point of ejaculation (point of no return), then paused, and, as soon as the arousal has dropped to a low level, the stimulation is resumed. This change between stimulus and pause is said to change the neuromuscular reflex mechanism and lead to an increase in the duration of an erection.

The "stop and start" method is almost identical to the squeeze technique discussed below. This method consists of sexually stimulating the man until he feels that he is almost reaching orgasm. The stimulation should be stopped for about 30 seconds and start again. Repeat this pattern until the man wants to ejaculate. At the last time, continue the stimulation until the man reaches orgasm.

Squeeze technique or pushing method

The squeeze technique consists of sexually stimulating the man until he recognizes that he is almost ejaculating. At that time, the final part of the penis (where the glans meets the axis) is gently pressed for several seconds. Stop sexual stimulation for about 35 seconds and start again.

The person or couple can repeat this pattern until the man wants to ejaculate. The last time, continue the stimulation until the man finally reaches orgasm.

Here the man learns to perceive his arousal and the time of the unwanted ejaculation more consciously. With this method, the penis should be pressed gently at the tip. As a rule, you put your index finger on the frenulum and your thumb on the glans and press lightly for several seconds. Shortly before ejaculation, the state of arousal usually decreases. After that, it is advisable to wait a few seconds to a minute and then resume sexual activity. Tip: Both the stop-and-start method and the push method usually require some training to make it work.

To do this, the penis must be stimulated through masturbation or sexual intercourse, and, when you feel that you will ejaculate, you must stop and put pressure on the head of the penis. You can do this by slightly placing your thumb on the underside of the head of the penis, above the bridle, and with your index and middle finger, press over the penis, enclosing the urethra. The pressure should be maintained for 4 to 5 seconds and should be slightly uncomfortable, but without causing pain.

This technique should be repeated a maximum of 5 times in a row. Another compression option is to tighten at the base of the penis. This technique can be done effectively during penetration, but it is important to ask the partner not to move, avoiding stimulation when making the compression.

Cool Draw Method

Cool draw method also called Testicle Breathing. Massage your testicles until you get a slight feeling of sexual energy. Now take a deep breath and simultaneously pull upwards using the muscles around the testicles and anus. As you do so, use your mind to visualize the sexual energy from your testicles being drawn out towards your anus. Then exhale slowly and relax. Repeat this breathing exercise a few times. While breathing, you should focus on the transfer of your sexual energy from your testicles across your perineum and towards the anus. You should eventually feel a tingling sensation moving across this path. Press your tongue once this happens, continue to breathe slowly and focus on that energy. Move it away from your perineum via the anus all the way up your spine.

You should be able to feel that tingling sensation moving through your body towards your head. It might take up to 10 minutes. But, eventually, the tingling will reach your head. At this point, you can press your tongue to the roof of your mouth and feel the energy slipping away down the front of your body. The whole technique is based around visualization and the use of the mind, as premature ejaculation, is often a mental problem. You can practice this technique several times until you begin to master it. Then, during sexual sessions, make use of it. This will help to draw the sexual energy away from your penis and testicles, freeing the pressure in these areas. Thus, allowing you to have sex for longer periods of time.

Masturbate before intercourse

This means getting busy before you "get busy." Many men report that they have better control over sex if they ejaculate beforehand. This affects younger men in particular. Because, with increasing age, many men have difficulty in building a new erection after ejaculation. The strategy is only suitable for men who can build a second erection after ejaculation in a certain time interval.

Strengthen your muscles: It is very important to know that weak pelvic floor muscles sometimes contribute to premature ejaculation. Kegel exercises can help to strengthen them. Find the right muscles to tighten, stopping your urine halfway. Hold them firmly for 4 seconds and then release them for 4 seconds. Always do this 10 times, at least 3 times a day.

Doing Kegel exercises

Kegel exercises allow you to strengthen the pelvic floor muscles, which are the group of muscles that are in the pelvic area and around the urethra. When these muscles get stronger, the man may probably be able to control ejaculation, preventing it from occurring when he contracts them.

The use of condoms to desensitize

The use of a condom can reduce sensitivity enough so that you can last longer. Some men experience that using a condom makes them less sensitive. By reducing the sensitivity on the penis, the ejaculation reflex is triggered later. As a result, many men have longer stamina. Men should try it out for themselves.

Taoists Natural Ejaculation Control Technique

Reverse abdominal breathing called Taoist breathing. In this method, the abdomen contracts inward during inhalation and relaxes outward during exhalation. This breathing technique is very effective for premature ejaculation, and it works your abs too.

Water

Cure Premature Ejaculation with Water. Water is a main component of the body. The lack of fluid in the body causes debilitating sexual function. Drinking more water can cure many diseases and also Premature Ejaculation.

Edging

Edging is a masturbation technique used for premature ejaculation. Masturbate until close to the point of ejaculation and stop the stimulation for a few seconds. Again start to masturbate and stop it on the edge of ejaculation. You can practice while doing sex.

Speed of Your Strokes

When you have sex, the same as the previous method leads to premature ejaculation. So you have to change the sex position, and also you should change your stroke speed (Slow stroke and fast stroke). Fancy the idea that you have to vary your stroke. You might try either of the following strokes:

- 10 slow stroke and 1 fast stroke
- 9 slow stroke and 2 fast strokes

Redirect thoughts before the climax

Some men believe that if they think about something else during sex, they can last longer. They try to distract themselves during the act and think about other things. This can also cause the sexual act to last longer.

Therapeutic measures by doctors or psychologists

Talking to a professional about the problem can also help. Some therapy sessions can help the patient reduce anxiety and find effective methods to avoid stress and work around problems. If these factors are resolved, the individual's sexual activity can significantly improve. These can also help reduce anxiety and frustration surrounding premature ejaculation. Sometimes there are other psychogenic factors, so that appropriate therapy makes sense here.

Sex therapy for premature ejaculation involves a few simple measures that are sufficient, such as masturbating an hour or two before sexual intercourse to delay erection during the act. Avoiding penetration for a while and discovering new sources of sexual pleasure can also be a way to take the pressure off penetration.

Physical activity with premature ejaculation

A new international study has shown that men with premature ejaculatio praecox may benefit from physical activity. Because it was found that men who are not particularly physically active suffer more from symptoms of premature ejaculation than physically inactive people. However, the study found no relationship between alcohol consumption and BMI in relation to premature ejaculation.

Various explanations were used. This includes that targeted physical exercises partially delay the reflex by activating the ischio-bulbocavernosus muscles in the pelvis that surround the penis. It was also discussed whether physical activity leads to a more positive perception of the body's image, self-confidence, and physical health, which in turn has an impact on sexuality. One should also not forget that so-called secondary ejaculation is often associated with incipient or already existing erectile dysfunction. Men who are not physically active are at increased risk of developing erectile dysfunction. And on the basis of this disease, secondary premature ejaculation can also occur.

Psychotherapy

Various psychological causes can be related to an EP, such as early childhood sexual disorders, unrealistic ideas about sexuality, fear of failure, and pressure to perform. Psychotherapeutic help can be used to break this spiral of fear. It may be necessary to involve the partner (talks and therapy), reduce anxiety, change thinking and behavior patterns, and reduce any sexual pressure to perform. Sex therapy, as well as behavioral, couple and family therapy, can be used to rethink behaviors and reduce anxiety.

The Glans augmentation technique

The Glans augmentation technique was originally developed to enlarge the male glans. The "positive" side effect: In patients who complained of premature ejaculation, the sensitivity of the glans was reduced after the procedure. The idea of using a filler like hyaluronic acid is now to create a barrier between the material used as the injection, the active stimulation, and the hypersensitive dorsal nerve receptors.

The hyaluronic acid gel is injected into the lamina propria. The thin layer of connective tissue lies directly over the nerve in the penis. This reduces the "emotional world" of the nerve receptors with tactile stimulation. The result of the intervention is not of an infinite duration because the hyaluronic acid is broken down again. The "barrier" is, therefore, not permanent lead to increased sensitivity in the area of the glans. If the nerves are completely severed, this generally results in a complete reduction in sensitivity. To build good erections, tactile stimulation of the glans is, of course, also necessary. A decrease in sensitivity could also lead to worse erections - up to erectile dysfunction.

MEDICAL THERAPY

The oldest form of pharmacological therapy is anesthetic ointments to reduce the sensitivity of the penis. By using special creams on the glans, this is reduced. Accordingly, some men report that they endure the sexual act longer before ejaculating. Background: In many cases, there is often increased sensitivity of the penis to touch and temperature in affected patients. The so-called biothesiometry provides information about this .

Medicines

Antidepressants can be useful because one of its side effects is to prolong the time needed to reach ejaculation. However, these drugs must be prescribed by specialists, such as urologists or psychiatrists. You can also apply a local anesthetic ointment to the penis to reduce stimulation. Decreased sensitivity in the penis can delay ejaculation. Using condoms can also have this effect on some men. If distraction techniques make it difficult to maintain an erection, medications used for erectile dysfunction can help.

Another option is to take so-called selective serotonin reuptake inhibitors (SSRIs) and tricyclic antidepressants, which were originally developed to change the state of mind. Studies have shown that these antidepressants delay the time until ejaculation, among other things. This side effect can also be used to treat ejaculation Praecox. Here, too, the man has to see whether the therapy is suitable for him. Dapoxetine is a short-acting SSRI for the treatment of ejaculation praecox.

Selective serotonin reuptake inhibitors (SSRIs), which are usually used for drug treatment, are the only approved drug in Europe from this group (dapoxetine) extends the time to ejaculation on average by only 1 to 1.5 minutes. Other SSRIs are significantly cheaper and more effective. They can be prescribed by the doctor as " off-label " treatment. The cost of medication to treat premature ejaculation is not reimbursed by the statutory health insurance, regardless of whether it is approved or not. This is because they are considered "lifestyle" drugs, and reimbursement for them is not legally possible. Drug therapy can take the form of gels or creams as well as tablets.

Medicinal topical (local) therapy is anesthetic gels and creams that are applied to the glans of the penis, reducing the sensation in men. There is also the **Medicinal (oral) therapy.** This involves the active ingredient dapoxetine used to delay ejaculation in the event of premature ejaculation by influencing the ejaculation reflex in the brain (oral therapy in tablet form). In addition, other medications can be prescribed, for example, if there is erectile dysfunction. The doctor will inform you about the use of other medications.

Only a doctor can tell you which medicine is best for you, as well as the correct dosage and duration of treatment. Always follow your doctor's instructions strictly and NEVER self-medicate. Do not stop using the medicine without consulting a doctor first, and if you take it more than once or in much larger quantities than prescribed, follow the instructions on the package insert.

Spray against premature ejaculation

Interestingly, European studies have shown that around 20 percent of men experience ejaculation within the first minute of penetration or shortly before penetration - this is known as "ejaculation antes da penetração." There are currently various therapeutic approaches to treat premature ejaculation (ejaculation praecox), for example, with a local anesthetic. This reduces the nervous information that occurs on the penis and is sent to the brain.

With Fortacin, a spray has been available since 2018 to prevent premature ejaculation and consists of a combination of the active ingredients lidocaine and prilocaine. The desensitization spray should be sprayed on the glans area at least 5 minutes before sexual intercourse. This reduces the sensitivity of the penis - at the same time, according to the approval studies, the time until ejaculation - increases by an average of 5.5 times.

There are a few points to consider before using Fortacin.

The spray should not be used if you or your sexual partner are allergic to any of the active substances mentioned. You should also be careful if you have ever had an allergic reaction to a local anesthetic. All other side effects should be discussed with the doctor or pharmacist in advance. Men with severe liver diseases, in particular, should avoid the spray.

If the spray comes into contact with mucous membranes, such as in the mouth or throat, a slight feeling of numbness can arise, which may reduce the sensitivity and the ability to feel pain. Fortacin must not be used together with other local anesthetics. And if condoms are used, which are made of polyurethane, for example, their effectiveness can be limited when using the spray - safe prevention of pregnancy or protection against the transmission of venereal diseases is no longer guaranteed. Before the sexual intercourse, 3 sprays, which corresponds to one dose, should be applied to the glans - within a day (24 hours) a maximum of 3 doses at intervals of at least 4 hours. In rare cases, the erectile ability is reduced by Fortacin. Some men are unable to build an erection despite spray and stimulation. A local burning sensation can also occur - by the way, also with the sexual partner.

MEDICINAL THERAPY AND ITS SIDE EFFECTS

Dapoxetine is a short-acting SSRI (selective serotonin reuptake inhibitor) for the treatment of premature ejaculation (ejaculation praecox). Scientific results and data from the patient's own group show that over 80% of the men who were prescribed dapoxetine did not continue the therapy in the first six months.

In an international study in which the average age of the patients was 38 years, all the men took 30mg of dapoxetine 1 to 3 hours before sexual intercourse. If they noticed that the 30 mg dose was not effective, they increased to 60 mg. A quarter of the men stopped therapy within a few weeks. 79% of all study participants discontinued therapy over a span of six months. After two years, over 90 percent of the study participants stopped taking dapoxetine.

The results coincide shows that the remedy is not effective enough, and the disappointment is big. Some men also report that they find it difficult to take dapoxetine 1 to 3 hours before the sexual act, as it cannot always be planned. A small proportion of patients reported that the intake was stopped due to side effects such as nausea or dizziness. In addition, dapoxetine is much more expensive than sildenafil, the active ingredient in Viagra, which is available on prescription for a few euros per tablet. The low effectiveness and the high therapy costs are, therefore a reason for many men to stop the therapy.

In the use of spray, to reduce the risk of distortion, such studies are usually carried out "double-bind," meaning neither doctors nor patients know who receives which medication. In addition, many clinical studies are placebo-controlled. In the studies with the new desensitization spray, IELT (Intravaginal Ejaculatory Latency Time) was measured - the time from penetration to ejaculation. Using the spray, the IELT increased on average from less than 0.6 minutes to 3.2 minutes. In the patients who were given a dummy treatment, the baseline values averaged 0.56 minutes, and the IELT was 0.94 minutes. The success of the spray can not only be expressed in numbers. The men participating in the study also indicated that their suffering had decreased significantly. In addition, they would have felt safer.

Before men use a desensitizing spray, the causes of premature ejaculation should always be clarified. Nerve changes, for example, can be identified by nerve measurements such as biothesiometry. In order to find effective therapy, other underlying diseases and disorders should also be clarified by the doctor. In addition to purely medicinal therapies, special mental training can also be very useful. Depending on the cause of the ejaculation praecox, the combination of both options usually produces the best results in the long term.

When using the desensitizing spray, but also the so-called local anesthetic creams (which, by the way, are off-label use and are therefore not permitted for the indication of premature ejaculation), men and their partners may experience a reduction in genital feeling. Genital hypoesthesia may cause women to have orgasm difficulties. And in some men, erectile dysfunction occurs because local stimulation is no longer sufficient to produce a sufficient, good erection. The bottom line is that there are many reasons that speak for and against the use of a desensitization spray. In any case, it is advisable to confide in an experienced doctor.

Hyaluronic Acid - Last Chance with Premature Ejaculation?

What is Hyaluronic acid?

Hyaluronic acid is multiple sugars and occurs almost everywhere in the body. In larger quantities, it is mainly found in the skin, but also in the bones and intervertebral discs, in the synovial fluid and in the vitreous of the eye. Hyaluronic acid is used as a medicinal active ingredient, among other things, for the treatment of joint wear (arthrosis). Because it is considered highly biocompatible, and it results in fewer physical reactions than a foreign agent. Wrinkle injection with hyaluronic acid is currently particularly popular.

How it might be your last step?

There are some patients who, despite good diagnostics and therapy adapted to the diagnostic result, still suffer from premature ejaculation (ejaculation praecox) . In the meantime, affected men have the option of reducing the sensitivity of the glans penis by injecting hyaluronic acid.

However, men should only consider this option as the last option!

The experts say: The American Urological Association (AUA) and the European Association of Urology (EAU) do not provide any surgical interventions for the therapy of premature ejaculation. The International Society for Sexual Medicine (ISSM) also speaks out against elective surgery of the dorsal nerve and the injection of hyaluronic acid. The point of view is based on the concern that there may be a permanent loss of sexual function because the sensitivity is extremely reduced. This should make men think who is considering taking this last step as a therapeutic measure.

Premature orgasm: Do women have it too?

In fact, women also get an orgasm before they want it - but rarely. Unlike premature ejaculation in men (ejaculation Praecox), however, female premature orgasm has not yet been adequately investigated.

However, scientists have found that around 39% of women have had premature orgasms. 14% of the study participants stated that this happens to them regularly; after all, 3% always have an early climax. A parallel: women do not feel particularly comfortable with an early orgasm - similar to their male sexual partners. In men, however, the premature coming means that he can no longer maintain the erection and, accordingly, there is no penetration. This is, of course, different for the female gender. Because women can continue sexual intercourse after orgasm, which many find uncomfortable. As with any sexual problem, affected women should contact a doctor they trust to take therapeutic measures if necessary. The treatment must be done in a comprehensive way, considering the various aspects of the patient and their context of life. Depending on the assessment of each case, drug and / or therapeutic treatment may be introduced. It is very important in this treatment the collaboration of the partner, being patient and transmitting security and confidence to the man.

HOME REMEDIES FOR PREMATURE EJACULATION

Erection occurs, basically, due to the directing of blood to the penis, which fills their cavernous bodies and provides support for the organ to become erect. Therefore, it is believed that foods that stimulate circulation may help in cases of premature ejaculation. However, as the problem is multifactorial, they are not guaranteed.

Garlic: Garlic has several interesting properties for health, including sexual. "It has anti-inflammatory, antibacterial, anticoagulant action, and aphrodisiac properties are also attributed to it. Its anticoagulant action improves blood circulation which can be reflected in the erection", considers the nutritionist Andreia Guarnieri

Saffron, ginger, and milk drink: Milk serves more as a base for this mixture, but the two spices have functions that justify being pointed out as home remedies for premature ejaculation. Saffron has great prestige as a sexual stimulant in the countries of the East, as it has a vasodilating effect, in addition to supposedly promoting increased sensitivity in the genital region. Ginger, on the other hand, also favors the circulation of the body, also helping to improve the quality of erections.

Rosemary sitz baths: Relaxation is essential for premature ejaculation sufferers, so the nutritionist Andreia believes that rosemary sitz baths can be a good home treatment. Rosemary is known to be invigorating, and sitz baths with fresh rosemary help to 'sedate' the genitals and promote physical and mental relaxation.

CHAPTER EIGHT

HOW THE FEMALE BODY WORKS

SEX ROLE VARIABLES

When we study the brain, we conclude that women generally approach sex differently than most men. Women want to be appreciated and desired, but above all, they want to be intimate. Sex is a means to increase intimacy for most women. The desire of a woman and the need for intimacy with a certain man arouses her desire to have sex with him.

Most women know that men who usually compete in all areas of work and play also have a desperate desire to be the best in bed. In most cases, women are less interested in PE than their partners. For her, sex is about love and intimacy, not ghostly sex, which is a very masculine point of view. Having sex does not necessarily mean sex based on an erection and focusing on penetration. Surprisingly, some couples find sex without penetration more exciting because they are looking for alternatives and do not repeat the usual habits of sexual intercourse.

On the other hand, most men achieve intimacy through sex. For them, intimacy is a happy by-product of sexual connection. A man's emotional reaction can include a sense of relief that he has not ruined everything. But most women who choose to have sex with a certain man are not there to judge him. You just want a special connection. Someone to share your intimate moments with.

We can conclude that men achieve intimacy through sex, while women need intimacy before and after sex. We can even come up with some behavioral generalizations:

Men strive for selfishness, while women seek meaning and relationships that lead to safety. While men can play with their willies when given a chance, women tend to look at sex more holistically.

In general, men are guided by sexual performance, and greater socialization does not help, but women judge sexuality based on feelings. Men wonder if this different concept of sexual satisfaction is the reason why women often need longer turn-on and cruise times to get to the point of not coming back. The extent of man's intimate dedication is more valid in the long run if done correctly.

Do men tend to sleep after sex, or do they switch to the sports channel? While women like to cuddle, talk, and stay together. So be aware of the different sexual functions and give her the intimacy she wants.

FEMALE BODY BASICS

Before we give you some tips on how to wake them up, let's examine some general facts about how your body works. Different women have different erogenous zones and orgasms. It is, therefore important to research your partner's unique body and communication. It may surprise you that not all women love their breasts. Most

121

women want to be touched everywhere, and it is the sensitivity of their touch in the less intimate areas (back, neck, face, arms, abdomen, around but not in the breasts and legs) that arouses their desire for touches your sexually sensitive areas such as breasts, nipples, clitoris and vulva. A good sign that she is on is when she starts pushing her vulva against you or gently pushing her hips into some kind of wave or wave motion.

Because they have menstrual cycles (and sometimes even afterward), women react differently to the body at different times. A woman's sex cycle depends on her hormones, which in turn determine how much she wants to have sex and how sexy she feels. Generally, the sexiest moments are immediately before and after menstruation. Some, for example, Willy volunteers, do not want to be touched at "Oprah."

The vagina is not always wet and ready to accept anything. If you don't wake up, your walls are relaxed and moving. The outer edge of the vagina, which is closest to the opening, is the most sensitive with most nerve endings. This includes

122

point G. Here's the hard part. Women with sensitive vaginal points (G or A) have them in different places in the vagina.

The size of your penis usually doesn't matter. Because the most sensitive vaginal areas are on the outer edge, more than size matters, and at least women fight for intimacy - a large penis alone doesn't cut it and can sometimes hurt. As with men, blood flows to all erogenous areas in excited women, and the vaginal walls exude a sweat-inducing fluid. Excessive vaginal lubrication does not always mean that she is very excited, and poor lubrication means that she is not switched on. It depends on the cycle and other mysterious female factors - let's keep a secret about how they work!

You may not be surprised to hear that women have no orgasm in most sexual encounters with men. Why do men usually come, and women don't? Nature's breeding plans may have something to do with it, but is it one of life's injustices? If we improved these statistics a little, the world would be happier. Not all women ejaculate with an orgasm like men. Some do, but there is debate about whether it is involuntary urine removal. Suffice it to say that most women do not ejaculate for our purposes.

For many women, orgasm is accompanied by pelvic contractions that you feel when you are inside. However, it is not for everyone, and only every woman knows whether she has come or not. Our eternal question: How do we know whether it really came or did so? Only she can tell you !!

Only she can give feedback that really tells you how good you were on the field. How well you managed to maintain and maintain the cruise period. An excited woman is one of the best experiences in life. There is a big difference in your experience of sexual encounters, depending on whether your partner is one or not. In addition, an orgasming woman will do wonders for her sexual experience.

They are also products from your past and, therefore, unique. So you have to spend some time understanding your Jane. Remember that you are actually doing this for yourself.

Now let's look at more anatomical facts about how they work.

THE CLITORIS

WHO IDENTIFIED IT?

Despite our thousands of years of fascination with the clitoris, it has only recently been fully identified. The anatomical analysis of the female genitals by Helen O'Connell, a urologist from Melbourne, showed that the clitoris is much larger than previously thought! Most are buried under layers of fat and are protected by the basin. The acorn of the clitoris is simply the much larger outer part of the body underneath. There is a body, two arms, and support lamps with lubricating glands! Let's look at a cross-section of a vagina with a "penis." The outer layers of the skin, fat, and muscles are disassembled and the penis is shown in position only in a simplified cross-section.

The upper end of the clitoris axis is exactly where these forks are located, above the woman's pubic bone. Between the pubic bone and the clitoris, there is a layer of fat and muscles that form a small pillow for it. A man's pubic bone is located just above the root of the penis and is also covered with a filling of muscle and fat.

We will review the components that make up the fascinating clitoris and play such a vital role in your response. To make it easier to identify the relevant parts with which we will try to relate, we start from what is visible above.

At the end of the clitoris, there is a sexually sensitive head called an acorn. You can call this the clitoris head. This glans has a foreskin or foreskin that retracts - just like Willy's foreskin. In most women, only the tip of the clitoris - the glans - is exposed, and only when the foreskin of the clitoris or the glans is pulled out and only when the foreskin of the clitoris is pulled out or when the clitoris is upright and from the foreskin.

Above the glans of the clitoris, usually, the only visible part outside the body, the body of the clitoris bends down and is called the arm of the clitoris.

This curve was also called the "clitoris knee." When you disassemble the outer layers of skin, fat, and muscle, the upper part of the shaft and glans look like a crooked little finger, with only the upper joint coming from the foreskin - a prosaic description of this fantastic part of women, the most of us prefer to write poems.

The body or stem of the clitoris bends down and divides into the two forks that surround the vaginal opening. At the end of the two forks, there are two lights - like Willy's balls. These veins and balls are made of tissue that is filled with blood during sex. It is believed that these lamps are part of the vaginal structure, but actually part of the erectile tissue of the clitoris. They seem to have a use. They transmit pressure from the vaginal mouth to the nerve structure of the clitoris and help close the urethra during arousal, which can prevent bacteria from entering the urinary tract during intercourse.

Let's say masculine. The glans (head) and shaft (penis) are connected, and the stimulation of both leads to an orgasm, although the stimulation of the glans probably leads to a faster orgasm. And just like a penis during sexual arousal, it has a kind of foreskin that retracts and makes the glans of the clitoris visible, but - and here it gets a little different - at the bottom of the two arrows on the clitoris are irritable. Interestingly (only to be observed), the glans of the clitoris retreat under the hood when stimulation is prolonged. This can be very surprising for us men because we wonder where it went. However, make sure that the stimulation responds even when it is not visible.

That is why the clitoris is fixed and full of blood, just like Willy, when he is awake. But it is also an advantage to have the clitoris repaired. Every pull on the shaft and forks of the clitoris during penetration is transmitted directly to the glans through the foreskin or the foreskin of the clitoris. So when a man walks in and out during sexual intercourse, his penis can pull and release the shaft and clitoris lamps around the vagina, creating the shaft and balls around the vagina, thus indirectly stimulating the clitoris glans.

However, such an orgasm is more difficult and takes longer than direct clitoral stimulation.

If the clitoris stands upright during sexual activity, it can grow longer, but it swells more and more as the curve above the glans flattens slightly, so that it shows a little less. The clitoris, therefore, has certain flexibility in this direction.

In addition, the branched axis is held in place by small inner bands that allow limited up and down movement in the centerline of the body.

Now there is more interesting news here. If two sexual partners have the same size, the same weight, and the same size and the same ratio of the legs to the upper body, the woman can position herself so that her clitoris is between the pubis and that of the partner. It is then possible for her to move during intercourse so that when the man stops his inner impulse, but just before pulling his penis out, the pelvis rolls down and out to properly squeeze the penis. Clitoris between the pubic bone. and their own. Again in the words of Catherine Yronwode: "So with each penis push the glans is rubbed along the filled pubic bone of his partner and the axis of the clitoris pulled down and then up. Clitoris - caused by the downward movement of the pelvis, which it ends up of the inner stroke of the penis - is the most pleasant of the two directions: the pelvis, the extent of the clitoral leakage can vary from one centimeter to one and a half centimeters.This applies not only to the missionary position but also to the woman at the top, which some women very exciting, lying on the man and he is quiet, without exerting pressure on the hip, she will be able to control the amount, regulate the pressure and the movement of the clitoris so that she adapts perfectly while she is I like how nice it is to practice our penetration exercises with her alone.

The Mysterious G Spot

A headline on SMH weekend editions reads: *"French slam Brits' G-spot finding."* Apparently, a British college recently found that the G-spot could be a myth. The French, who did not accept British authority over sex, responded at a conference that denounced the foolish Britons looking for genes: "I think their Protestant, liberal, and Anglo-Saxon character means that there has to be a reason for everything, one gene for everything ... and that's why they have to question everything because they can't find a G-spot gene. "During the Dr. Foldes (French) conference that not all G-points are the same. Foldes (French) has indeed claimed that not all the G-points are the same. He even said that the very sensitive area has little resemblance with the famous magic button that is guaranteed to provide instant pleasure. They (the French) concluded that the G-spot could only be felt by women who know that it exists and took steps to cultivate it Sylvain Mimoun (French) added: "If she never played ... there won't be for her".

For some of us, with partners who have found and cultivated it, here is how a woman deals with her G-spot: "I think this is not the place to investigate how or why a small point in the Vagina is a woman works as a channel for huge reserves of sexual and spiritual energy! Believe me, this place has something special that goes beyond our understanding and gives us access to another dimension of sexuality. "I think we all agree that we should know everything about G-Spot. Well, almost everything. Willy, who retired from a teenager, was looking for a GT streak.

Who identified the G Spot?

In The G Spot and other recent discoveries about human sexuality (by Alice Ladas and others), the authors claim that the German obstetrician and gynecologist Ernst Grafenberg (the original Mr. G himself) has already described a feeling zone along with the submarine - the urethral surface of the anterior vaginal wall. He also concluded that there is always an erotic zone along the course of the urethra on the front wall of the vagina, which appears to be surrounded by erectile tissue such as the erectile tissue cavity of the penis. It should be noted that the term "G-spot" was not used by Grafenberg itself. As mentioned above, he called it an "erotic zone," which is a much better description of it.

How do you find it?

133

Willy reappeared, but I think we can ignore his suggestion that you find a G-spot with a mechanical device. The rest of us can make it worse than listening to a smarter scientific opinion for a minute or two.

I hope nobody passed out. To find the G-spot, insert a finger into the vagina (it is polite to ask first) and move it over the top wall of the vagina while the woman lies on her back with her legs apart. In the upper vaginal wall, there is a piece or two of tissue that is clearly different from the rest of the vaginal wall. You can describe the G-spot as a very soft area, an inch or two in the vagina on the top wall.

When you try this for the first time, it is a practical trick for the man to touch the woman as he lies down next to her, palm over the clitoris, fingers bent down, and into the vagina. If he bends his finger as if calling someone, the G-spot must start to respond and the woman can become ecstatic.

If you are looking for an orgasm at the G-spot, you have to try different movements: pushing, rubbing, pushing, and everything at different speeds until you find the best. Since all women are different, you need feedback from her about what works better and feels better. Don't forget to start slowly and increase your pace as it drives you more. Our clinical team can confirm that it is particularly satisfactory when performed with oral clitoral stimulation.

What about the G during intercourse?

During sexual stimulation, the female urethra and G-spot swell and swell and become soft and soft. It is easy to feel. The urethra grows in width and length and pulls on the cervix (a natural reflex to protect the neck wall against Willy's blow). Natural sweat provides delicious lubrication. At the end of the orgasm, it swells strongly.

As your excitement diminishes, it becomes more difficult and flashy. In order for an orgasm to occur at the G-spot, the G-spot usually has to be flexible, relaxed, and swollen. It is this elevated trajectory that, according to Grafenberg, "is a primary erotic zone that may be more important than the clitoris." He explains that its meaning was lost when "mission position" became a dominant characteristic of human beings when "mission position" became a dominant characteristic of human sexual behavior. Other sexual positions stimulate this erogenous zone much more efficiently and thus cause vaginal orgasms.

CHAPTER NINE

FOOD & DIET FOR A HEALTHY SEX LIFE

One of the main reasons for the problem of premature ejaculation is the increased acidity in your body. This acid in your body is caused by metabolic waste, which in turn largely depends on your diet. Some food products produce acidic metabolic waste and therefore increase the acidity of the system, while others produce basic metabolic waste and therefore reduce the acidity of the system. All of these staple foods help you, and keep problems under control, while those acidic food bodies increase the level of acidity in your problem and exacerbate your problem. -

I will give you a very simple and clear example. Baking powder is of basic nature and is usually food-grade, meaning it can be taken immediately. Take 1/4th of a spoonful of baking soda and mix it well with a glass of water. Mixing this in water, it was easy in nature. Drinking this water after about an hour of consumption not only helps you get rid of heartburn (many people have the problem of acid, heartburn, etc. when eating spicy food in the pan) meal) also helps you cope with the PE problem. It has direct effects and works within a few hours. It can be used as home remedy. For many of you ,dapox prong and dapoxetine have the same effect as a 60 mg dose of this home remedy and can be taken about two hours before sex. Although I don't suggest that you use this trick very often, it can be only be used occasionally. I will work better that way and more naturally.

This example of sodium and its effects clearly show the importance of controlling this "acid" in the body in PE problem. You have to exclude all acidic products from your eating habits. In general, all processed foods are naturally acidic, for example, bread, pizza, etc. Similarly, all fried foods are naturally acidic. All sweets, cold drinks, soft drinks, juices packed with sugar syrup, etc. are inherently acidic.

Pickles are also acidic in nature. This list is not exhaustive, but you can use these general guidelines to help you decide which foods are basic and which are acidic. You would generally reduce these foods from your diet. Milk tea (black tea and green tea can be taken without added sugar) and coffee should be avoided entirely. These two drinks not only increase the acidity in your system but also your weak nerves. Weak nerves cannot give you strength. Everything, which is difficult to digest, is probably the acid in your system. Spicy food is difficult to digest and increases your problem. Most non-vegetarian foods also fall into this category.

Everything, what raw, untreated, and easy to digest, the rule is simple in nature , such as salads, sprouts, fruits, boiled and steamed vegetables, etc. The less cooked food, the better is it. You need to incorporate more and more of these items into your eating habits for better results.

Based on the above principles, I give my customers the following tips. These tips work wonders, and you should definitely give it a try. Even if you don't get results with these tips, be patient and continue to follow them through the discipline feed that I said above, they will definitely show their effect in due course.

Start your day with "sprouts." Including Brussels sprouts for breakfast. Every sprout is sufficient. Whichever one you can easily get and organize, it's enough. A small bowl is enough. Common snouts (Cicer arietinum or Gram or Chana) and mung beans (Vigna radiate or Moong or Gram green) are easier to shoot. You just have to eat them raw.

Dip Chana or Gram (Cicer Arietinum) in a bowl of water overnight . Drink this water in the morning. You
can also eat this chana soaked, raw, or with salad

or vegetables or in any other way. It's a trick that's really helpful for getting rid of PE.

Make it a habit to chew a spoonful of fennel teal (saunf) after each meal. Fennel seeds have various health benefits. Among other things, it can also offer improved hair and clear skin. It helps with the digestion of food and is basically simple in nature. It will cure your indigestion and acidity. Within a week, its effect on showing its increase in strength and retention is noticed.

Here are a few mix, boost, and teas prepared in the form of remedies from readymade materials that will improve your retention and help you fight premature ejaculation:

Almond mixture

This remedy is called "turbocharging" because of the long-lasting hardening it offers the penis muscles. The almond mixture guarantees sexual expansion and a long-lasting erection. Almonds are very good in too rapid ejaculation to avoid because the brain and nervous system to feed, to improve their function. The almond is very rich in vitamin E, calcium, potassium and minerals, proper sexual function, and energy men released to promote. Increases the release of a high amount of testosterone, which increases libido. Almond also acts as a recipe with two fronts, provides the energy for sex, is needed, and receives the libido in men upright, causing the sexual performance is improved. Nutmeg in honey increases sexual desire and helps the erection of the penis to support. The combination of the chemical onion gives a strong fragrance, is responsible for increasing blood flow to sexual organizations, making sexual desire, and prolonged erection increases. Saffron is a mild natural aphrodisiac

Recipes

- 2 tablespoons of ground almonds
- White onion
- ginger powder
- 200 g pure honey

- 2 tablespoons of nutmeg powder
- Powdered cardamom
- turmeric powder

Steps

- Cut onions and mix in pasta
- Pour the honey into a pan.
- Add 2 tablespoons of powdered almonds and onions.
- B Borrow the nutmeg powder and add two tablespoons.
- Add a teaspoon of ground ginger
- Add half a teaspoon of powdered cardamom
- Add a pinch of turmeric
- Stir the contents well
- Heat for 5 minutes.
- Let the pasta cool
- Drink a cup every morning and feel an improvement in sexual performance

Mix of garlic

Garlic is one of the most effective means of treating premature ejaculation. The effectiveness of garlic cannot, because of the overestimated be content of allicin very high in garlic. Allicin promotes an increase in blood flow and strengthens the blood vessels in the penis, which means that the penis prolonged erection can be maintained even after ejaculation. This is a characteristic of garlic, which makes it a preferred recipe for erectile dysfunction treatment. Garlic contains antioxidants that detoxify the body and aphrodisiacs that optimize sexual performance in men.

Recipes

- 5 cloves garlic
- Indian buffalo butter - 2 tablespoons

Steps

- Add 2 tablespoons of ghee to the pan and heat over low heat for 2 minutes.
- Add the ghee 5 garlic gloves and stir one minute long to.
- Let the mixture cool.
- Eat once every morning.

The tonic increases healthy sexual performance and keeps the erection longer and prevents rapid ejaculation. This remedy is your penis erect even holds after ejaculation and allows you to instantly have sex a second round, with no interest to lose.

Pomegranate Boost

Several studies carried out into the use of pomegranate in the show effectiveness of the treatment of erectile dysfunction and the in-state of life without a good time to ejaculate. However, the result of the most significant therapy with pomegranates i s expanded with the use achieved. Pomegranate also lowers blood pressure.

Recipes

- ¾ cup of milk
- pomegranate seeds
- Strawberries - 1 liter

Steps

- Place the pomegranate seeds in a clean bowl with a liter of strawberry.
- Put in a blender and stir until smooth. You can also use a juicer to achieve this.
- Sift the juice into a glass.
- Add the milk.
- Mix well.
- Drink a cup of pomegranate juice daily. It must also be taken between 30 and 45 minutes before sexual intercourse. This is, however, works at best, when in the morning with the intention, the sex in the same evening.

Asparagus mixture

Asparagus is a plant, since ancient times in the treatment and the treatment of erectile dysfunction, premature expulsion is used and the maintenance of sexual health. It is a very powerful natural aphrodisiac, in which the male potency increased, and the male libido increased

Recipes

- Honey - 4 tablespoons
- asparagus leaves
- Milk - 200 ml

Steps

- When the asparagus goes and puts it in a pan.
- Enter 200 ml of water into the pan and heat the asparagus 5 minutes long.
- Pour the liquid part into a cup of tea
- Add 50 ml milk
- Add 3 tablespoons of honey
- Take this medication twice a day, especially before sex.

Ashwagandha Boost

Also known as ashwagand, it is an adaptogenic tonic that helps in stabilizing psychological processes
and promotes homeostasis. It helps reduce
stress, a major cause of erectile dysfunction , and premature

ejaculation. Ashwagandha contains functions that the increase of energy increases the resistance and allows the penis to erection for a long time, so the maintenance of sexual desire.

Watermelon is a very important part is the mixture "Viagra-like" sustenance called the rich citrulli to keep the blood flow in the penis during intercourse.

Recipes

- Honey - 2 tablespoons
- Ashwagandha dry seeds
- 200 ml of milk
- watermelon

Steps

- Put the milk in a saucepan then heat for 3 minutes
- Grind the dried ashwagandha seeds into powder.
- 3 tablespoons of honey .

148

- In 2 teaspoons of ashwagandha powder.
- Add half a glass of water
- Add watermelon juice along with the seeds
- Mix well.
- Drink a glass twice a day.

Tamarind mix

Tamarind contains natural properties that include: male fertility, sexual capacity, increases the initial appetite, treat dysfunction, erectile , and ejaculatory. He has an endurance test.

Recipes

To prepare
Tamarind mix, are these recipes requires:

- Tamarind seeds.
- 3 teaspoons of pure honey

Steps

- Remove the tamarind seeds and dry them.

- Grind the dried seeds into powder.

- Put 2 tablespoons of tamarind powder in a glass bowl.

- Pour hot water over the tamarind powder into the glass and let it cool.

- Drink a glass twice a day. This triggers your sexual response and prevents you from ejaculating on time during sex.

Arugula Erectile Boost

Arugula, also known as rocket salad, contains properties that make it a very powerful aphrodisiac. It blocks contaminants that can reduce sexual desire. It has a high content of vitamins, calcium, and magnesium. The arugula increases the blood flow to the blood vessels in the penis and thus supports the erection of the penis. It helps youthful vigor and energy to keep during sex.

Recipes To prepare Arugula erectile boost, the recipes are:

- Arugula leaves
- 200 ml of water
- G powder - 1 teaspoon
- 3 tablespoons of honey

Steps

- Put 200 ml of water in a kettle and heat for 5 minutes.
- Wash and mix rocket
- To give arugula juice into a cup of tea. Pour the hot water into a cup of tea.
- Add 1 teaspoon of ground ginger.
- 3 teaspoons honey too.
- Drink a glass twice a day.

Mustard seed remedies

Mustard seed is another very important means of treating sexual dysfunction. It contains circulation-promoting properties. Good blood flow leads to good sex because the penile erection is determined by the amount of blood that circulates through the blood vessels in the penis. The penis is made up of muscles and blood vessels, so anything that prevents proper blood flow to that part of the body will result in a weak erection. The banana was added to this remedy because it contains bromelain, which causes the production of testosterone and prevents premature ejaculation. Pine nuts are very rich in zinc, which is essential for healthy sexual desire.

Recipes

To prepare Mustard seed remedies, the following recipes require:

- 1 gram of mustard seeds
- 200 ml of water - honey
- 2 tablespoons of ginger powder
- 7 ripe bananas
- 1 tablespoon of pine nuts in powder form

Steps

- Dry mustard seeds and grind to a powder.

- Take a bowl with a lid

- Put 200 ml of water in the bowl.

- Add 2 tablespoons of mustard powder

- Add 3 tablespoons of honey

- Add 2 tablespoons of ginger

- Peel and mix the banana.

- Add the banana juice. Add 1 tablespoon of powdered pine nuts

- Stir contents, put in a pan, heat for 2 minutes, and let cool.

- Drink 20 minutes before sex.

Solid rock boost

Rock Solid Boost is a basic therapy for a longer erection period during sexual intercourse. It is very easy and quick to prepare at home. It also improves the quality of the sperm produced in the testicles and increases fertility.

Recipes

- 1 tablespoon of ground ginger
- 80 g cabbage
- 90 g celeriac
- pomegranate seeds
- ½ teaspoon of cinnamon powder
- 400 ml of water
- 2 tablespoons of honey

Steps

- Pour 400 ml of water into a clean pan.
- Add 110 g of cabbage and heat
- Cut the celeriac into medium sizes and put in the pan
- Let the 20 minutes of cooking and let cool.
- Extra ct pomegranate seeds in a blender
- Put ½ teaspoon of cinnamon powder in the blender.
- Pour the cooked cabbage and celery TOG root ether with the water that is kept cooked in the blender , the pomegranate seeds, and mix until it is pressed.

- Strain to the solution, to obtain only the liquid content in a glass, and with 2 tablespoons of honey on .

Oat straw tonic

Oat straw, also known as Avena Saiva, is rich in vitamins, minerals and induces serotonin secretion in the brain. Serotonin relieves stress, anxiety, improves the dilation of blood vessels in the genital area, increases sexual interest in men getting an erection during sexual intercourse for a long time upright, increases immunity, and helps to calm the nerves. Oat straw is in the first place is considered as a natural mood stabilizer that empties the mind, a tonic for sexual potency, because it increases sexual interest and helps premature ruptures occur in males. If a man during sexual intercourse quiet is , is the tendency , to the last longer and maintain a strong erection is greater than when it is stressed or anxious. Studies suggest that anxiety and stress primarily responsible for libido are and , in most cases, to cause premature ejaculation. Oat straw tea is, therefore, a very important tool in the treatment of sexual dysfunction with years of positive results.

Recipes: For this remedy, the recipes are as follows1 ounce of dry oat straw

- 2 tablespoons of pure natural honey
- 200 ml of water

Steps:

- Crush powdered oats.
- Boil 200 ml of water in a kettle
- Take a jar with a lid
- Put 2 tablespoons of oatmeal powder in the glass
- Pour the boiling water into the pot over the straw of the oat and stir.
- Cover the pot and let it stand for 10 minutes
- Pour the liquid content into another cup of tea. Discard residues.
- Add 2   tablespoons of natural honey Add to sweeten   the tea. Avoid the   use of granulated sugar because sugar starches   not

only destroy crystallized herbal tea, but eating too much sugar is a major cause of premature ejaculation during intercourse in men.

- Stir well and drink a cup three times a day.

CHAPTER TEN

ULTIMATE EJACULATION MASTERY

The best approach to learning the ultimate Ejaculation solution is what I called the RAMPER, which means:

- Relaxing
- Awareness
- Monitor your level of arousal
- Pacing yourself
- Energy circulation
- Ride on the wave

I will familiarize you with the most important aspects of each topic so that you know how to perfectly practice it.

Relax

Do you remember what normally happens to our bodies when we reach climax? We tighten and contract our pelvic muscles, especially on the buttocks, anus, stomach, and legs. What do you think will happen if your muscles were completely relaxed while you were really excited? You probably wouldn't come. This is a simple technique, but it takes a bit of practice to learn. After six years of practice, I finally got very good at it. Sometimes, everything you need to do to prevent you from enjoying stands inside and outside of you. That's why relaxation is an important feature of Ultimate Ejaculation Solution. Why? It is calm and relaxed because the ideal condition enables you to do just that. Tension blocks blood flow and affects feelings, not to mention the flow of orgasmic energy that is associated with that. When your channels are blocked, your energy collects in the genital organs.

As there is no place to go, you feel more and more under pressure to ejaculate. The energy searches for the path of least resistance beyond the top of your vajra. If you don't want to come, open the inner channel and let the energy rise through the inner flute, you can replace the rush more easily every time taste sensations want to make you peak. Normal sex session, on average, is much slower than the fast pumping you see in porn movies. By going slowly, you are more relaxed. How do you learn to relax while excited? First,   do   your best to eliminate stress during sexual

encounters. A lot of tension arises from fear or uncertainty in the implementation. If you can get out of your head and just enjoy the moment, you'll find it much easier to relax. This often requires communication and partnership with your loved one. Because therein lies your head, expectations about to have are what will happen and how you want it to occur. THINKING ABOUT SEX is always worth less than actually having sex.

Getting out of your head means letting go of so many worries that are usually associated with sex, even with long-term partners. Setting mental goals   can work   for   you   in business good work. But when it comes to dealing with internal energy, it can work against you and distract you from living the moment. The ultimate solution to ejaculation, as contradictory as it may be, is to ignore the need to control the outcome of your sexual act. Your goal is to enjoy and relax. Once you've learned to be relaxed, comfortable, and passionate about the natural flow of juicy energy, you'll enjoy flying instead of losing it.

You can relax by performing "Solo Exercises" regularly with physical techniques that will help you relax mentally. The most important of these relaxation techniques is breathing. Do you remember what happens to your breathing when you come? They soon begin to and panting breath. What do you think would happen if you knew how to breathe deeply and slowly even though you were flooded with ecstasy? You made it, and you would be washed inside and out with orgasmic energy, without much stress.

Awareness

If you are considering bringing your partner to their own ejaculation, orgasms will consume your awareness. The ultimate ejaculation solution helps to produce incredibly mutual orgasms without much need for concentration. As previously reported, you need to focus on the pleasure at this point. If you know how well your Vajra is now, you are more likely to be willing and able to relax. When you and your partner make love, stop every now and then and just feel how good it is. For you to focus pleasure, you should reasonably increase your focus. That means alignment in all senses: taste, touch, sight, sound, and smell. It means enjoying every view, enjoying every fragrance, and enjoying all sensations. If you become more sensitive to everything that happens in your body, you will not have the usual situation of untrained lovers: total concentration on the sexual organs.

Instead, you can spread this wonderful energy across all of your chakras. As mentioned earlier, you can arouse relaxation on your senses and , at any time to embrace the sensations. If you have not learned the power to follow the moment without goals or expectations, mental stress will draw your attention to the feelings of the moment. Most importantly, most of us who come too quickly are not very good at recognizing the internal signals that can warn us of impending ejaculation. If you learn to register all the little nuances of all the little feelings, walk slowly and digest all your energy, you are less likely to stumble across the point of no return, and consequently enjoy sex in its essence. When you enjoy every breath, every sound, and every movement, you are very aware of your own tension. And you will be able to on this excitement respond before it is too difficult to manage them, by pushing on the cliff and plunge into the abyss.

How can you control your energy flows if you are not fully attuned to them? Then you cannot. Make it your mission to you to focus on your feelings. To enhance your senses, emotions, enjoy the fun without a book, and you will gradually come out of your head, and bring your body to come when you actually want to.

Monitor your level of arousal

At this point, you've heard over and over that you need to tune your senses and sensations. What are you doing with this keen awareness? M in RAMPER means to monitor and measure your excitation level. This is not just a scientific experiment, but a method that makes you more sensitive to what inspires you. If you know where your excitement is and what is causing it, you can play spontaneously while increasing your excitement and that of your partner. Then you can take responsibility for your own pleasure, the act of the leaders of love, so you really excited and remains there without too far to go. Arousal awareness is complex, very subtle. It's more like a rainbow than black and white.

The forces that excite us are not always clear at this point and change from time to time. So step

M is about learning to read from yourself, so you know exactly where you are. Many sex therapists recommend using a 10-point scale to monitor your level of arousal during exercise and during sex. This is one of the most important things we will focus on in the following exercises.

Pace yourself

OK, you have relaxed. You have become a bit less sensitive. You measured how good it is. Will this   change your resistance drastically? Well, yes, or maybe not. But the RAM part of the PAMPER technique is simply vital preparation for the P. P means to Pace yourself along the way. No, I'll take it back. P stands for pleasure. If you focus on pleasure and not on orgasm, you won't suddenly come across a goal. You don't finish in a race. You have no schedule to meet. You just slow down and enjoy the moment. This is a big part of the pace. And if you learn to make the fun, you enjoy greater than a quick dribble you have ever experienced, and you will need more, more and more!

We'll talk later about partners who are so excited they won't leave you in a hurry. Of course, that happens, and in an onslaught of orgasm, they drag you across the abyss. And if you enjoy it together like that, it's a great moment! But when it comes to pushing, most enthusiasts want you to be through all night. Then you will finally hear the reason with the right kind of guidance. I will then show you how ecstatic participation can apply to you. The ultimate ecstatic solution is to learn to walk on the edge, this fine line between absorbing all the fun and consuming and enjoying it at the same time. For this reason, as I said, I am rarely heard talking about total control. Control makes you stiff, tense and stiff, which is the total opposite of relaxation.

Control requires that you set patterns and watch yourself all the time and stop the flow of energy to get off the threshold. The idea of pacing yourself is relaxed, more like jumping from one wave to another than the surf struggling maneuvers and many large throttle adjustment struggles. Relax, enjoy the sweet sensations as you ride the wave, and gradually and carefully add a little tension as you take the wave. The key to "P in Pace Yourself" are the other two more P-words with peaking and plateauing. The charms adjust cause sudden excitement waves so that you return, without limit to be   exceeded. If you represented a summit, it would be a steep climb and a steep descent. There he got this name. Plateau is the advanced skill that you learn when you sleep well in spines are.

Plateau is about learning at a high level of excitement maintenance, without having to go backward. Now, do you see what relaxation, awareness, and measurement will do for you? These are the essential tools you use to detect when you reach a point that comes very close to the point of no return. With this increased sensitivity, you can stop quickly at this moment

Energy circulation

E means energy, and it circulates away from your genitals. But it can also mean Ecstasy. You can even think about Ultimate Ecstatic's solution over SEX teach what Subtle Energy Ecstasy is. Since most are programmed from forward, to seek the Big O from the get-go, we enter the arena of a love game and are often tempted to release our sexual energy by explosive sexual genital. It is what is glorified in books, films, and conversations in the locker room. This is the accepted concept of good sex in most people's minds. Who among us is lucky enough to be introduced respectfully and openly into the higher dimensions of sacred sex? Few if any, at all. So here is an essential part of your initiation; your happiness lasts. Instead of shooting at Big O, increase your energy around and through your body while your arousal increases, so you have even more pleasure.

Some say it will supply your brain with cosmic energy and give you psychedelic visions. However, you should know that you will not only be amazed, but because you are not consuming your energy, you can last way longer. How you do that? Simply put, you channel your sexual energy into the inner flute of your first chakra (the sexual center at the base of your spine) so that your little Willy's head doesn't explode in a stream of ejaculation. You send your orgasmic energy mainly through the four pillars of presence, breathing, sound, and movement. Admittedly, learning may not be as easy as describing it. It will certainly take months. Make you the right as it is when the excitement of the Vajra for pulsation brings and takes up other parts of your body. It reminds you of the first time you've tried that, that is to draw energy from my genitals, without exploding. If I could experience this awesome experience, so could someone else.

Therefore, the E of the RAMPER is to channel your orgasmic energy elsewhere in your body. Where you going, and what are you doing? Well, first, it moves in your heart and energizes your love center. Do you know how women always shout when they meet a sensitive man? You will love it if your heart is activated by sexual energy. And when one of your chakras is actually activated, you can flood your partner's corresponding chakra with your energy. The current energy becomes an exercise of sharing bliss and pleasure within you. You'll need the four orgasm keys - presence, breathing, sound, and movement - to strengthen your energy and feel more passion. These are the main tools of the circulating energy - visualizing the juice spreads inwards, breathing deeply into the abdomen , moaning with pleasure, shaking hips and squeezing the sexual muscles - pumping the energy into the internal whistle.

After practicing for a long time, I really proved that expressing love sounds like releasing energy that would otherwise get stuck in your genitals. It may take some getting used to. But it's worth it, in the end. Believe me, your partners will love to hear how excited you are. As discussed above, the net effect of learning to just ride the moment helps to separate the ejaculation orgasm. If you relax inside and remain super excited, contractions around the prostate to initiate ejaculation will not be activated. When the energy gets intense, you can still have those strong pelvic contractions that are quite great for overall excitement. This leads to a dry orgasm, a long series of pleasant and slow cramps, without ejaculation and with a wave of energy. I call this "implosive orgasms" because the energy is pumped back and forth. The best news for you is when you have a dry implosive orgasm, your arousal suddenly drops dramatically. And on the other side of this climaxing, you will suddenly be less sensitive and relaxed. So you quickly put up your Willy and build up emotions slowly again.

Ride the Orgasmic Wave

If you keep your inner energy, your pleasure rises higher and higher. That is why the abbreviation RAMPER is so appropriate and describes how your pleasure   does increases. Those of you who enjoy sex rapidly will never experience these growing plateaus. This means you have never developed your ability to take in more and more pleasure. When you finally do that, it will feel like waves of ecstasy are coming right from within you. The ultimate solution is really ecstatic when all the parts are pieced together? Relax, and you will increase the awareness of your ability to open subtle energy. By creating excitement to measure, you learn how to walk to the top and mount the plateau.

This collects an intense amount of energy within you, which circulates the whole body, rather than exploding in rapid ejaculation. Then bring up the shaft, and you just hover. If you up to your energy to your spiritual centers, the upper chakras rise, and you'll have a natural feeling of peace and happiness all around you. It will be is as if their energy orgasmic was the psychological nature feeding his soul. That's why we call it tantric sexual meditation. Some describe it as a hollow bamboo, with an endless energy supply, through your body between the earth and the air flows. Tantric Sex uses the same body parts and erogenous zones that you see in X-rated movies, but the actions inside and outside are very different. Tantric lovemaking, both mentally and physically, is slow and conscious.

It's not only about an orgasm, but about giving pleasure to oneself and making it last like forever. This requires harmony, openness, and a lot of communication between the partners. As you get more and more comfortable with the same partner, there is no doubt that you experience movements and tips that indicate when to use them. Even the most experienced lovers cannot always predict the moods and changes that occur in spontaneous lovemaking. Therefore both partners have to be coordinated. This only works if you receive verbal or subtle instructions from your loved one. Tantric love partners are really a team, fully synchronized. But if you are single and trying to find a partner, or if you have a completely different experience, the type of orgasm wave I just described can cause problems. I'm good at orgasm, but when I'm in contact with a wilder partner, which is not in sync with me, I will come soon. There are different types of enthusiasts, and we are not all compatible with each other – that is why sexual compatibility is very important.

CHAPTER ELEVEN

FREQUENTLY ASKED QUESTIONS AND ANSWERS ON
PREMATURE EJACULATION

Here are a few questions and answers to round up our whole discussion and improve your knowledge about Premature Ejaculation. Some of them have been answered in the chapters preceding, but they are deemed important enough and needed another shout out for reinforcement.

1. After all, what is premature ejaculation?

The new definition came out of a consensus involving experts from around the world. The group divided premature ejaculation into two categories: primary and secondary. "In the primary, prematurity happens since the beginning of sexual relations and the time elapsed from vaginal penetration to ejaculation is less than one minute," explains urologist Luiz Otávio Torres, from the International Society of Sexual Medicine and one of the authors of the guideline. In the secondary type, the man had no complaints about his performance between four walls, but, for some reason, he starts to expel the semen faster than he would like - he does not reach three minutes of sex. For you to have an idea, the global average (and considered normal) is around five minutes.

2. Is it normal to ejaculate faster after many days without sex?

Yes, it is natural. And it happens for physiological reasons (the accumulation of sperm) and because of the wait to have sex with the beloved. "The individual mentalizes the scene in advance, and they will only grow," says urologist Mariano Barcelos Filho, from Hospital Mãe de Deus, in Porto Alegre. For this reason, experts suggest masturbation to anyone who will stay away from their partner for long periods. In return, things tend to unfold without much haste. There is a study that correlated sexual frequency and ejaculation. And the result was that the withdrawal time could influence the control of ejaculation, yes.

3. If the penetration time is only short sometimes, is there an indication of a problem?

The latest edition of the Diagnostic and Statistics Manual for Mental Illness, DSM-5, from the American Psychiatric Association, reports that to be diagnosed, the disorder must be repeated in 75% of sexual relations. "It is necessary that it persists for more than six months," adds Carmita Abdo, coordinator of the Human Sexuality Studies Program at the University of São Paulo (USP). If the failures are sporadic, they are related to stress and other momentary issues and do not deserve specific treatment. There is also no drama if the boy is in his first sexual experiences.

4. Do circumcised men have less premature ejaculation?

Circumcision has nothing to do with premature ejaculation. Removing the foreskin, the skin that covers the head of the penis does not seem to have much influence on the time of sex. "Circumcision should be encouraged more for a hygienic reason," says Barcelos.

5. Would using a condom help, as it reduces the sensitivity of the penis?

Yes, the strategy works for some men, because the condom imposes a barrier that reduces the contact of the penis with the vagina. "But the studies that evaluated its effectiveness in this regard are not conclusive," counters Sidney Glina, urologist and professor at the ABC Medical School, in Greater São Paulo. In the big guys who claim to benefit from the strategy, thicker latex models are preferable. It is worth remembering: despite the problem, putting on a condom is an indispensable tactic to prevent diseases and unwanted pregnancies. The condom can help with treatment, as it can decrease sensitivity and delay ejaculation. In addition, there are condoms with medications that decrease sensitivity and lead to a delayed ejaculation effect.

6. Home techniques, like thinking about bad things right now, work?

On the internet, it is common to find very creative solutions to delay ejaculation. One suggests that a man thinks of something boring when he feels he is about to come. But you can't take the hint to the letter: being discouraged in such an exciting context decreases the loving interaction with the partner and even ends the erection. One way out would be to give the glans a strong squeeze seconds before ejaculation, as the pain would lessen the rush. "It works, but it is important to understand and cooperate with women," recalls Miguel Srougi, professor of urology at USP's Faculty of Medicine.

7. And enjoy quick oral sex? Is it premature ejaculation?

Scholars have not found enough evidence to format concrete definitions of premature ejaculation for oral and anal sex. "The consensus was restricted to vaginal sex," confirms Glina. For the time being, it is not possible to stick to what is premature in other modalities.

8. Does drinking alcohol delay ejaculation?

Yes, because drinks relax and soothe anxiety. But this is a dangerous path: the man can gain a dependency on beer, whiskey, and the like to have a satisfactory sexual relationship. And then, if you can't drink anything.

9. Does the position influence the time of sex?

It depends on the couple. Generally speaking, positions like Dad and Mom and on all fours excite the man more, since they mainly require his movement. With muscles of hips, pelvis, and legs contracted, ejaculation tends to come fast. "The least stimulating positions are him with his body on his side or with his partner on top," exemplifies Carmita.

10. Who takes time to have an orgasm need to worry?

Although rare, the disorder exists. It is anorgasmia caused by antidepressants, low testosterone, or emotional instability. Psychotherapy and drugs solve the situation.